STUDY GUIDE

for

Pharmacology for Canadian Health Care Practice

Second Canadian Edition

STUDY GUIDE

for

Pharmacology for Canadian Health Care Practice

Second Canadian Edition

Linda Lane Lilley, RN, PhD
Scott Harrington, PharmD
Julie S. Snyder, MSN, RN, BC
Beth Swart, BScN, MES

Study Guide prepared by
Julie S. Snyder, MSN, RN, BC
Adjunct Faculty
Old Dominion University
Norfolk, Virginia

Beth Swart, BScN, MES
Daphne Cockwell School of Nursing
Ryerson University
Toronto, Ontario

With special thanks to
Linda K. Wendling
for her contribution to the first edition

Study Skills by
Diane Savoca
Coordinator of Student Transition
St. Louis Community College at Florissant Valley
St. Louis, Missouri

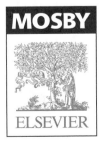

MOSBY

ELSEVIER

MOSBY
ELSEVIER

NOTICE

Knowledge and best practice in this field are constantly changing. As new research and expertise broaden our knowledge, changes in practice, treatment, and drug therapy may become necessary or appropriate. Readers are advised to check the most current information provided (i) on procedures featured or (ii) by the manufacturer of each product to be administered, to verify the recommended dose or formula, the method and duration of administration, and contraindications. It is the responsibility of the practitioner, relying on their own experience and knowledge of the patient, to make diagnoses, to determine dosages and the best treatment for each individual patient, and to take all appropriate safety precautions. To the fullest extent of the law, neither the Publisher nor the Authors assumes any liability for any injury and/or damage to persons or property arising out of or related to any use of the material contained in this book.

The Publisher

Library and Archives Canada Cataloguing in Publication

Study guide for Pharmacology for Canadian health care practice / Linda Lane Lilley ... [et al.] ; study guide prepared by Julie S. Snyder, Beth Swart ; study skills by Diane Savoca. – 2nd Canadian ed.

ISBN 978-1-897422-64-9

1. Pharmacology–Canada–Problems, exercises, etc. 2. Nursing–Canada–Problems, exercises, etc.
I. Lilley, Linda Lane II. Snyder, Julie S. III. Swart, Beth, 1948- IV. Savoca, Diane
V. Title: Pharmacology for Canadian health care practice.
RM301.P4564 2010 Suppl.   615'.1   C2010-900590-2

Vice President, Publishing: Ann Millar
Managing Developmental Editor: Tammy Scherer
Publishing Services Manager: Jeff Patterson
Senior Project Manager: Clay S. Broeker
Proofreader: Jerri Hurlbutt
Cover: Gopalakrishnan Venkatram
Cover Image: © doc-stock/Corbis
Typesetting and Assembly: SPI Publisher Services
Printing and Binding: Transcontinental

Elsevier Canada
905 King Street West, 4th Floor, Toronto, ON, Canada M6K 3G9
Phone: 1-866-896-3331
Fax: 1-866-359-9534

Printed in Canada

1 2 3 4 5 14 13 12 11 10

Student Study Tips

TIME MANAGEMENT

Time and money have much in common. They can be spent, saved, invested, given away, stolen, and wasted. The big difference between these two commodities is that you can earn more money, but your time is limited. Learn to manage your time now and the quality of your life will increase because you will have more time to do what you enjoy.

You may not enjoy studying. What you want is to be a nurse, but studying is one choice that will get you what you want. Being a nurse will bring you the satisfaction that you need. I, for one, am very thankful that you have made this decision. The world needs dedicated skilled nurses. To meet this need, you must make the decision to manage your time effectively.

GENERAL GUIDELINES
Establish Goals and Create Action Plans

One key to time management is having clear goals and an action plan to accomplish these goals. This is more than saying, "I want to be a nurse" or "I want to ace my pharmacology midterm." It is a decision to spend time now to get clarity and direction so that you will have more time later to relax. The following guidelines can help you get what you want.

Guidelines for Setting Goals

There are some basic guidelines to follow when setting goals:
- **Be realistic.** The goal must be something that you can reasonably expect to accomplish. A goal of scoring 100% on each and every unit test is not realistic, but a goal of scoring 85% or better is.
- **Be specific.** Goals must set out exactly what needs to be done. Do not simply state, "I will study for the exam." Specify how many hours, what days, and what times you will study. The more specific the goal statement, the easier it is to establish a plan, complete that plan, and thus achieve the goal set.

- **Establish a time limit.** Specify a time limit for completing each step in the plan and an overall deadline for accomplishing the goal.
- **Make the goal and actions measurable.** State the goal and each step in the plan for achieving it in a way that will enable you to measure your progress toward completion.

The following is an example of how this goal and action process works: You have a chapter test a week from today. The test will cover approximately 45 pages of text material, and there are 40 specific pharmacological terms you must know. In addition, you have been given about 20 pages of supplementary handouts in class. What will you do in the next 7 days to prepare for this test?

Goal statement:
I will study to make a good grade on this exam.
This is a poor goal statement because it is not specific, sets no time limits, and offers no real way to measure progress. The intent is good, but the implementation of such a vague goal is usually poor.

Revision 1:
I will spend 2 hours a day studying for the next chapter test in order to get at least an 80% score.
This is a better goal statement. If one assumes that 2 hours per day is realistic, then the goal is more specific, the grade goal is measurable, and there is a time limit of sorts. This goal statement might be good enough, but it could still be improved.

Final version:
I will spend 2 hours per day, from 2:30 to 4:30 P.M., for the next 7 days studying for the chapter test in order to score at least 80%.
This is what is needed. This version states how much time, when, how many days, and for what purpose. Setting clear goals helps you get started and serves as a motivator to keep you working.

Guidelines for Action Statements

A goal, no matter how well stated, is not enough. There must be action statements to help you make day-to-day progress toward meeting the goal. The guidelines that apply to defining your goal also apply to establishing the action statements—they should be realistic, specific, measurable, and time limited. They spell out what is going to be done day to day. Here are three examples of good action statements for the sample goal:

- I will master six pharmacology terms each day.
- I will spend from 2:30 to 3:00 P.M. each day reviewing class handouts.
- I will review 10 pages of text material from 3:00 to 4:00 P.M. each day.

These examples should give you a good idea of how to go about developing a clear goal and a set of actions to carry out to achieve that goal.

Organize Tasks and Create Schedules

It takes time to make time. It is your choice. Either you set your schedule or others will do it for you. It is 2:30 P.M. The phone rings and friends want you to go out or your boss wants you to work overtime or your sister wants you to watch the kids. When you have an action plan and a schedule, your choices are clear. This is the time you scheduled to review class handouts. Can you reschedule this review or do you want to keep this promise you have made to yourself to accomplish your goal? No matter what you decide, you have maintained control over your time.

Your goals and action plans are the foundation for your time management. The next key is to organize tasks and create schedules.

Guidelines for Organizing Tasks

1. Divide tasks into three categories:
   a. Jobs that **have to be done,** such as going to class, going to work, eating, and getting adequate rest. These jobs are the easiest to accomplish because the consequences of not doing them are serious. If you do not go to class, failure is almost a sure thing. If you do not go to work, soon there will be no pay-check. The consequences of not eating or sleeping are obvious.
   b. Jobs that **should be done,** such as studying, cleaning, and all of those other necessary but unpleasant tasks that are part of life. The "should-be-done" jobs are the most difficult to accomplish because they are the jobs that are all too easy to put off doing. These are also the jobs for which time management skills are most essential.

   c. Things that you **want to do.** These include all of the fun things that provide pleasure and escape from the routines of class, study, and work. Most of us are successful at finding time to do what we want to do, even when there is a siz-able backlog of "should-be-done" chores waiting. This choice can lead to procrastination and stress. The important things are maintaining balance and staying focused on your goals.

2. Prioritize items in your **"have-to-be-done" category** based on your physical and mental health needs. Examine the consequences of not doing these activities. If you can live without doing an activity, then it is not a need.

3. Prioritize your **"should-be-done" category** based on your physical and mental health needs. Examine the consequences of not doing these activities. Can you accomplish your established goals without doing a given activity? If so, then it is not a need.

4. Prioritize your **"want-to-do" category.** Some recreational time is absolutely essential in any effective time management system. "Want-to-do" activities can often be used as incentives for completing what should be done.

5. Use incentives to accomplish what you should do. For each person the rewards will be different. Spend a little time determining what will work for you. It might be watching your favourite reality show, prime time drama, or comedy show; going to the movie theatre to see a new release; reading a book for pleasure; or just spending some time with family or friends.

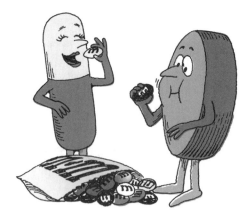

Guidelines for Creating Workable Schedules

You will need three types of schedules: **master, weekly,** and **daily.**

Start by developing a **master schedule** table on your computer that has 7 columns and 15 to 17 rows. The columns are the days in the week and the rows are the hours in the day. The left-hand column will represent Sunday and the far right will be Saturday. Start at the top of each column with the time you usually get up in the morning and end each column with the time you usually go to bed. A typical master schedule might begin at 6 A.M. and end at 11 P.M.

Once the blank schedule sheet is prepared, the next step is to fill in those hours that correspond to the activities you have to do. These are the hours others control, and the activities are those that occur at the same hour, on the same day or days, and for several weeks or longer. For example, the semester's schedule of classes is the first set of activities to enter into the master schedule. Other activities such as work, travel, worship services, and any other regular activities also belong in the master schedule.

The master schedule should contain only those recurring activities that cannot be done at any other time. Activities such as doing the laundry, watching television, and shopping should not be included, because the time when you do them is more flexible. The idea behind compiling the master schedule is to establish those times of the day that are "spent" and therefore cannot be used for any other activities. The empty blocks that remain represent the time you have to do everything else. Figure 1-1 shows a sample master schedule.

Creating a master schedule takes no more than a half-hour, and it will generally serve you for an entire semester. The only reason to compile a new master schedule is that a significant schedule change has occurred. You may get a new work assignment or your nursing practicum site may change and require an additional 15 or 20 minutes of travel time. Then a new master schedule should be drawn up to accommodate the increase in time that is now necessary. Once the master schedule is completed, make four or five copies of it. These copies will be used to prepare the detailed weekly schedule.

Next, move on to developing your **weekly schedule.** The master schedule helps you identify the time you have available to complete the **"should-be-done"** and **"want-to-do"** task lists. The weekly schedule is more complex. It is intended to help you plan for study, recreation, family time, and all those other activities that you want to fit into a typical week. To prepare the detailed weekly schedule, take one of the copies you made of the master schedule and begin to fill in activities in the open blocks of time. The first blocks of time you should assign are the most important ones for any student—study time. This is what time management is all about—scheduling the needed hours of study (Figure 1-2 on the next page).

When filling in study hours, consider these important factors:

- **Amount of planned study time.** There is an old rule pertaining to study time, and even though it is an old rule, it is still a good guideline. The rule is to plan 2 hours of study time for each 1 hour spent in class. For example, a three-credit-hour course meets 3 hours per week, so you need to plan 6 hours of study time per week for this course. Remember, this is a general rule. Some courses will not actually require as much

	SUN	MON	TUES	WED	THUR	FRI	SAT
7:00		GET UP		GET UP		GET UP	
8:00		TRAVEL		TRAVEL		TRAVEL	
9:00	GET UP	CLASS		CLASS		CLASS	
10:00	CHURCH	CLASS	TRAVEL	CLASS	TRAVEL	CLASS	
11:00	CHURCH		PRACTICUM		PRACTICUM		
12:00		CLASS	PRACTICUM	CLASS	PRACTICUM		
1:00			PRACTICUM		PRACTICUM		
2:00		PERSONAL	PRACTICUM		PRACTICUM		
3:00		PERSONAL					
4:00		AEROBICS		AEROBICS		AEROBICS	
5:00							
6:00		DINNER	DINNER	DINNER	DINNER	DINNER	
7:00							FUN
8:00							FUN
9:00							FUN
10:00							FUN
11:00	BEDTIME	BEDTIME	BEDTIME	BEDTIME	BEDTIME	BEDTIME	FUN

▼ **FIGURE 1-1.** The master schedule. This is an essential first step in managing time effectively.

	SUN	MON	TUES	WED	THUR	FRI	SAT
7:00		GET UP		GET UP		GET UP	
8:00		TRAVEL		TRAVEL		TRAVEL	
9:00	GET UP	CLASS	*STUDY*	CLASS	*STUDY*	CLASS	
10:00	CHURCH	CLASS	TRAVEL	CLASS	TRAVEL	CLASS	*STUDY*
11:00	CHURCH	*LUNCH*	PRACTICUM	*LUNCH*	PRACTICUM	*LUNCH*	STUDY
12:00		CLASS	PRACTICUM	CLASS	PRACTICUM		*PERSONAL*
1:00		*STUDY*	PRACTICUM	*STUDY*	PRACTICUM	*STUDY*	PERSONAL
2:00	*FREE*	*STUDY*	PRACTICUM	*STUDY*	PRACTICUM	*STUDY*	PERSONAL
3:00			*TRAVEL*		*TRAVEL*		
4:00		AEROBICS		AEROBICS		AEROBICS	
5:00							
6:00		DINNER	DINNER	DINNER	DINNER	DINNER	
7:00	*STUDY*	STUDY	*STUDY*	STUDY	*STUDY*	STUDY	FUN
8:00	*STUDY*		*STUDY*		*STUDY*		FUN
9:00	*STUDY*	*REVIEW*	*REVIEW*	*REVIEW*	*REVIEW*		FUN
10:00							FUN
11:00	BEDTIME	BEDTIME	BEDTIME	BEDTIME	BEDTIME	BEDTIME	FUN

▼ **FIGURE 1-2.** The detailed weekly master schedule. Fill in the study times first.

time as you allot, whereas others will require more. The reason for beginning a semester with this approach is simple. It is easy to find things to do with time you do not need for study, but once a semester is under way it can be very difficult to find additional study time. If you do not plan enough study time at the beginning, you will soon find yourself in a constant battle to keep up. The result is frustration, anxiety, and a sense of impending doom—feelings you do not need when you want to perform at your best.

- **Personal prime time.** Do you wake up early, ready to charge forward, but find it difficult to be productive after 10 P.M.? Do you do your best work in the afternoon and early evening and prefer to sleep until 10 A.M.? Are you a night owl? Answers to these questions will reveal your prime time, those times of the day when your ability to concentrate is at its best and you can accomplish the most. These are the times you want to use for study. It is not always possible, because of class and work schedules, to schedule all study time in your prime hours, but it is essential that those hours be used for study as much as possible. It would be foolish to plan to study your toughest material between 9 and 11 P.M. when you know that is a time when just reading the daily paper is a challenge.
- **Study hours for specific courses and general study hours.** The reason for scheduling both general and specific study times is that the study demands of

different courses vary from day to day and week to week. For instance, you will need some hours of study every week to master new material, terms, and concepts in pharmacology, but the study time demands will increase in the days just before exams, midterms, and project due dates. The hours set aside for specific courses are for accomplishing the day-to-day study demands; the unassigned study hours are for meeting the changing demands posed by these special circumstances. These unassigned study hours also let you meet unexpected demands. No matter how carefully you plan your time, something will happen to prevent you from using the time block you had set aside for learning.

Be patient and evaluate what works for you. It usually takes two or three attempts over a period of 3 weeks to arrive at a detailed schedule that works well for you. There is a tendency on the first attempt to try to schedule some important activity for every waking hour. Ultimately such a schedule will make you feel as though there is no time for fun. Determine what is not working for you and make appropriate adjustments. Each week your schedule will come closer to being realistic and effective. The need to evaluate and revise is the reason for making several copies of the master schedule. Or you may want to use an electronic calendar. It saves time in the revision process, and saving time is, after all, what time management is all about.

Your last scheduling activity is to create **daily schedules and lists.** No matter how carefully and thoughtfully you prepare the detailed weekly schedule, it cannot include all the tasks you will face. You will have small tasks, infrequent tasks, and unexpected tasks that will need to be added to your schedule. Each day as you think of things you want or need to do the next day, it is easy to either write them down (carry a small notebook that will fit into a pocket or purse) or make use of scheduling technology and input tasks into a handheld electronic device such as an iPhone, Blackberry, Palm Pilot, or PDA (personal digital assistant). Many devices offer calendar, memo, or task reminder features and allow users to organize a daily schedule that can also be synchronized to a desktop or laptop. The schedule can be reviewed regularly and revised as priorities change.

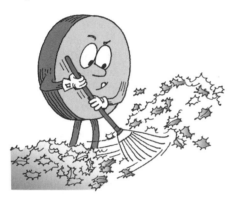

Consider the following when setting priorities:

- **There are only 24 hours in each day.** Be realistic about what you are able to accomplish. Do not plan to review three chapters of text material on a day when you know there will not be enough time to cover more than half of one chapter.
- **Everything is not important.** Rank your tasks as A, B, or C, with A being the most important and C being the least important. Then go about completing your As. Procrastinating about your B and C lists is not a sin. For example, going to the dry cleaners is critical if the outfit you must wear tomorrow is there, but if you do not absolutely have to have that outfit tomorrow, then the trip to the cleaners is a low priority and can be postponed to another day. Then it will be on your A list.
- **Rewriting to-do lists can steal your time.** You may want to make one weekly list and mark the tasks as A, B, or C. Put only A tasks on your daily to-do list. If you have extra time you can look at your weekly list. Or you can keep your tasks on note cards and then each day stack them in priority order.
- **Planning your route can save you time.** Look at the small tasks listed, such as picking up milk

and dog food, dropping off dry cleaning, and going to the bank. Not only plan to do those errands but also think about the order in which they should be done. Planning your route so that it completes a circle from home to the cleaners to the grocery store to home will be much more time efficient than going from home to the grocery store, back home, then to the cleaners, and finally back home again.

- **As you complete a job on the daily list, cross it off.** Crossing it off tells you that you are making progress and motivates you to move to the next item on the list. If not every item is crossed off, remember that tomorrow is another day. Celebrate what you did get done and create a plan for tomorrow that will help you accomplish your goals.
- **Remember your goals and planned action steps.** When unexpected daily tasks push them onto the B list, be sure to revise your plan to get back onto your time line. Put planning on your A list.
- **Waiting time can be a gift.** Small blocks of time are often lost or wasted because it does not seem as though anything significant could be accomplished during them. If you learn to use these small blocks effectively, you can free up larger blocks for more time-consuming or fun tasks. If a class ends 10 minutes early or if you are waiting for your ride, use the time for study. Take advantage of such "found" time to review five vocabulary terms, rework a set of class notes, or preview the next five pages of assigned reading. Using the odd minutes in the day to your advantage can really help you achieve your goals as a student.

Your time is a valuable resource for you to manage or to waste. The choice is yours. Stop for a few minutes and think over the previous strategies on how to manage your time: establishing goals and creating action plans, organizing tasks, and creating schedules. Which of these strategies will you choose to apply?

CHOOSE TO USE YOUR RESOURCES

This Study Guide is one of the resources that will help you be successful in this course. When you choose to apply these study tips, they will help you to be successful in all of your course work. Three other resources are your textbook, your instructor, and your classmates.

Your Textbook

The authors of your textbook have taken great care in organizing the information provided in a manner that will assist your learning. Each part starts with study skills tips that build on the tips that are presented in the Study Guide. At the beginning of each chapter, you will find specific objectives describing what you are expected to know and be able to do as a result of studying each chapter. Each chapter also contains learning activities and a glossary of terms. Take 10 minutes right now to perform a survey of your textbook so that you know what to expect over the term of this course. Look for chapter titles and Points to Remember. Later in this Study Guide you will find tips for mastering your textbook.

Your Professor/Instructor

Your professor or instructor wants to hear your questions because this demonstrates that you are interested in learning and are actively engaged with the material in your textbook and lectures. The instructor is an expert on the content and the type of tests that will be given in the class. Ask questions about what will be covered on a test and the type of questions you can expect. Office hours are designed to make your instructor available to you. Choose to get your money's worth and use them!

Your Colleagues

We all have different learning styles, strengths, and perspectives on the course material. Participating in a study group can be a valuable addition to your nursing school experience. These groups can be a fun way to learn. Teaching others helps us to learn and aids in organizing the course material. A study group is made up of students who are in the same class and who want to learn by discussing the course material. There are guidelines for organizing successful study groups.

1. Carefully **select members** for your group.
   - Choose students who have **abilities and motivation** similar to your own. Socializing and gossiping can eat up valuable study time. Noncommitted and underprepared classmates can be a drain.
   - Look for students who have a **common time to meet.**
   - Select colleagues who have **different learning styles** from yours. They might understand the reading material or lecture material better than you. They may be able to draw a diagram that will help your learning.
   - Find students who have good communication skills—people who know how to listen, ask good questions, and explain concepts.
2. Clarify the **group's purpose and expectations.**
   - Where and when will you meet?

- How often will you meet? How long will the meetings be?
- How much individual preparation between meetings is expected?
3. **Exchange names, phone numbers, addresses, and e-mail addresses.** Have a plan in case of emergencies.
4. **Plan an agenda** for each meeting.
   - Put the date and goal for the session on the top.
   - List the activities that will help you accomplish the goal.
   - At the end of the study session, list the results of your efforts and set the date and time for your next session.
   - Make assignments for the next session.

There are also some useful strategies to follow:
1. Exchange lecture notes and discuss content for clarity and completeness.
2. Divide up difficult reading material and develop a lesson to teach the information to each other.
3. Quiz each other by turning objectives at the beginning of each chapter into questions.
4. Use the Critical Thinking and Application and Case Study sections in this Study Guide as a basis for discussions.
5. Create and take your own practice tests. Discuss the results.
6. Develop flash cards that review key vocabulary terms.

This list could go on and on. Work with your group to design the strategy that works for you. Each study group you work with will be different.

Often in career programs like those in nursing, medical, and law schools, the course study group will turn into a learning group. **Learning groups may meet over several semesters even when the members are not taking the same classes.** Learning groups help you to prepare for licensing examinations, laboratory work, clinics, or practicum experiences. They focus on understanding and application in the field.

CHOOSE TO DEVELOP YOUR VOCABULARY

Participating in study groups and learning groups is an asset when you are working to develop a new vocabulary. Every specialty or discipline has its own language that must be learned for full mastery to occur. When you learn vocabulary with a group, you can hear others using the terms and they start to become real to you. Courses such as this one on pharmacology contain extremely complex material, and terminology is a major component of that complexity. As you learn to integrate this vocabulary into your discussions of the discipline, it will seem less like a foreign language. In technological, scientific, and medical areas, mastering the vocabulary can make the difference between being successful and struggling constantly to understand the ideas and concepts being presented. It is therefore helpful to adopt some strategies that can make the process of vocabulary development easier and more effective. Working with a study group is one strategy, but there are several more.

Use Dictionaries

You must have a good current reference dictionary. A desk reference dictionary is a hard-bound dictionary and not a condensed or paperback version. *Current* means the most recent edition of whatever dictionary you choose. A dictionary published 10 or 15 years ago may contain most of what you need, but unless there have been periodic revisions, as shown on the copyright page, it is almost certain to lack some information, and this may cause you problems. Alternately, electronic dictionary subscriptions or credible online medical resources and dictionaries such as MedlinePlus provide quick access to current and relevant information as well as definitions.

Reference the Text Glossary

As soon as you look at any of the chapters in this text, you will discover the glossary. A glossary is nothing more than a text-specific dictionary. It contains the terms and definitions the authors consider essential for a full understanding of the material. The glossary will not necessarily contain every term that is unfamiliar to you. (This is why you need a good dictionary.) You can begin the process of mastering vocabulary by paying particular attention to the glossary and key terms.

Create Flash Cards

Obtain a supply of note cards. Pick the size that best accommodates your handwriting style and size. If 5″ × 7″ cards do not fit into your notebook, pocketbook, or book bag and this discourages you from carrying them around with you, then use 3″ × 5″ cards. Remember, the flash cards these become are one of the best things you can study on the run.

Use What You Know

When you encounter an unfamiliar word, do not automatically assume that you have no idea what it means. Use the knowledge you have already acquired in other nursing courses and throughout your life.

For instance, *psychotherapeutic* appears in the chapter title for Chapter 16. Your first reaction may be that you do not know what this term means. By using what you know, however, you may be able to make an educated guess as to the meaning of the word without consulting either the text glossary or a dictionary.

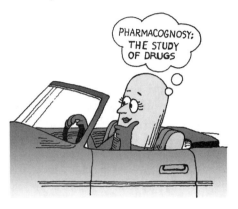

This is how you make that educated guess. Consider that the first part of the word is *psycho*. By this point in your career as a student, you know that *psycho* refers to the mind. This is a good start. Now consider the next part of the word. The meaning of *therapeutic* may or may not be evident to you, but it should remind you of a simpler word, *therapy*, which is the treatment used to cure or alleviate an illness or condition. Put *mind* and *treatment* together, and it would seem that *psychotherapeutic* must refer to the treatment of mental problems.

Note that this is an educated guess. It may not be a perfect definition, but it will give you a basis for acquiring a fuller understanding when the term is defined in the glossary or introduced and defined in the text of the chapter. The first sentence in Chapter 16 confirms that this educated guess is very close to the actual meaning: "The treatment of emotional and mental disorders is called *psychotherapeutics*." Using this approach to analyzing the meaning of a word not only confirms that you have a basic understanding of the word but also cultivates a mental link between what you know and the more specific definition provided in the text. Words and their meanings learned in this way are usually easier to grasp and easier to retain. Unfortunately, this technique will not work with some of the terms used in pharmacology because they are so specialized and specific to the field. This calls for the use of other techniques.

Learn the Standard Abbreviations

Make sure as you read that you pay attention to the "shorthand" used. For example, in Chapter 13, the abbreviation *CNS* is used repeatedly. The first time it is presented, the authors identify it as standing for *central nervous system* by putting the abbreviation in parentheses after the term. Thereafter, the abbreviation is used in lieu of the long term. The same thing is done for *REM* in this chapter. It is essential that you learn these abbreviations and recall each, not as a set of meaningless letters but as a key term that must be mastered.

Establish Relationships

REM is an abbreviation for *rapid eye movements*, and this term refers to a particular stage of sleep. Chapter 13 deals with CNS depressants. Relating REM to the focus of this chapter will help you remember that CNS depressants are used to influence sleep. The idea is to establish a clear relationship between the terms used and the ideas presented. Words should not be learned in isolation from the material; otherwise, you may know a lot of words and their meanings but not be able to relate them to ideas and content. *On tests, you are not likely to be asked just to repeat memorized definitions.* Instead, you will be asked to integrate these meanings into your answers to questions about nursing practices and applications.

Another important way of relating words to meanings is to link the meanings of closely related terms. The words *hypnotic* and *sedative* are good examples of this. In looking at the meanings in the glossary, you will find that each refers to a certain class of drugs. Both classes of drugs influence the CNS, but the drugs in each class have a somewhat different effect. It is useful to start with the understanding that both affect the CNS but then to appreciate how the terms relate to each other. Sedatives inhibit the CNS but do not cause sleep; hypnotics at low dosages have the same effect, but at higher dosages they may induce sleep. In this learning method, you learn meanings by looking at the general similarities and then at the specific differences between terms. In doing this, you have learned both words and should never have any problems relating the words to their meanings.

CHOOSE TO TAKE EFFECTIVE LECTURE NOTES
Why Take Notes?

The primary reason for taking notes is to help your memory. It is impossible to remember everything that is said during a 1- to 2-hour lecture. The act of writing something down helps strengthen learning and memory. In addition, note taking helps to focus attention on the lecture. It is easy to take mental vacations during a lecture; note taking helps keep you involved.

Note-Taking Problems
1. **Selectivity** is the biggest challenge. How do you know what is really important?
2. **Unfamiliar vocabulary** causes confusion. This is particularly true in a course heavy in technical, medical, and pharmaceutical terminology such as this one.
3. Hard-to-read or even **illegible handwriting** is frustrating.
4. It is **difficult to listen and write at the same time**. It splits one's focus and often gets in the way of understanding.

Note-Taking Solutions
1. Realize that note takers are made, not born. You can learn to be more effective as both a note taker and note user, but **this requires some practice** and a willingness to adopt new techniques.
2. **Use the vocabulary development** strategies previously discussed so that you will have a better understanding of the lecture material.
3. **Note taking is a five-stage process** that is spread out over the days and weeks between lectures and the time when you are reviewing your notes in preparation for a test.

Stage 1: Be Prepared

Note taking begins before the lecture. Read assigned material before class. This provides you with the background needed to listen intelligently to the lecture and to be selective when taking notes. You will have less unfamiliar vocabulary. The lecture will bring the textbook content to life for you.

Go to class a few minutes early and review your notes from the previous lecture. This will help warm up your brain so it will be ready to receive new information.

Stage 2: Active Listening

Taking quality class notes requires active listening. This is one of the most challenging aspects of being a good note taker. It requires an awareness of both the lecturer's language and nonverbal style. You have to pay attention not only to what is said, the verbal aspect, but also to the visual, nonverbal, aspect of the presentation.

Active listening requires selectivity. If you spend the lecture time trying to write down every word, you will not be able to listen to and therefore grasp the ideas. Focus on the most important ideas, terms, and facts to be recorded for later review. Writing less and listening more is a good rule to follow for note taking.

Learn to listen for key words and phrases. These vary with the subject content and with the individual lecturer, so there is no way to provide a single, definitive list of them. However, there are some verbal signals (words) that will give you clues that the lecturer is about to give important information:

- Sequence words—*first, second, next, then, last, finally*
- Contrast words—*but, however, on the other hand*
- Importance words—*significant, key, main, main point, most important*

The use of words and phrases such as these is the lecturer's way of signaling the relative importance and progression of certain facts and ideas. As important as these words are, however, it is also necessary to be aware of the volume, tone, and pace of delivery. Some instructors will slow down or repeat ideas that are important. Other instructors may speak louder and point into the air to emphasize a point. Get to know your instructor's style and you will be able to anticipate what will be on the test. Of course, if the instructor says, "One of the most important drugs in the treatment of…," then you should immediately know that what follows is an important point for your notes. The instructor has even told you it is important. As you practice active listening and observing in the lecture environment, you will find that your ability to discern the important ideas will improve.

Stages 1 and 2 are preparation for the real work that goes on in the last three stages.

Stage 3: In-Class Note Taking

The split-page note format requires a change in the way you set up your note paper. In this method, each sheet is divided into two parts by drawing a line down the full length of the page to create a left-hand column that is 6 to 8 cm in width and a right-hand column that is 14 to 15 cm in width. The right-hand column should be used for taking class notes. (The function of the left-hand column will be explained in the description of Stages 4 and 5.)

There is no magic formula for note taking. Simply take the best notes you can. Remember, notes are personal. Do not judge your notes against those of other classmates. Some will take a lot of notes, and others with a different background and expectations will take far fewer notes. The key point is to do what works for you. When what you are doing stops working, then try another strategy.

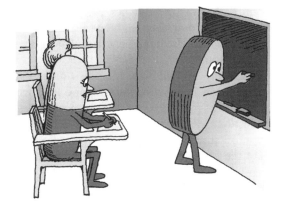

Here are some tips for taking effective lecture notes that may make the process easier and more effective for you:

- **Write in your own words** most of the time. Writing ideas in your own style will make them easier to learn and remember.
- **Leave space** between main points. When you sense that the lecturer has moved to a new idea, leave a couple of lines blank on your note paper. That way, if the lecturer returns to this point later, you will have room to add further notes. Even if there is no need for additional notes, the blank lines will help you see the organization of the ideas and the relationship between them. This space can also be used to add information that is from the textbook.
- Indicate **direct cues** from the lecturer, such as "This will be on the test," "This is a difficult concept," or even "Know this." Put a star or a check in your notes so you will remember to study this information when preparing for the test.
- Be especially aware of the **visual presentation**. This consists of information written on the chalkboard or presented using an overhead projector, slide projector, Power Point display, or other electronic display. Many lecturers outline key points on the chalkboard as a means of staying focused on the points they want to cover. Use this information to help you stay equally focused. Electronic displays are often chosen because the ideas can best be understood when they are presented visually.
- The **repetition** of certain points is the single most useful tip that they are really important. When an idea, term, or fact is important, the lecturer will almost certainly repeat it. For instance, the lecturer will introduce a new term, define it, give a couple of examples to clarify the definition, and finally redefine the term. This repetition is a signal that it is very important for you to learn the information.
- Be alert for **questions directed to the class**. These questions are another way the speaker stresses important information and are also a way for

him or her to find out how well the students have understood what has been said. Such questions are thus also cues that certain information is important.

- Be **actively involved** in what is going on in class. This means being willing to respond to a question directed to the class. It also means asking questions when things are not clear. Do not feel that because no one else is asking questions you are the only person who does not understand something. It is highly probable that there are others who are just as confused. Your objective in class is to understand the lecture and record key ideas in your notes so that you can study effectively. Questions are not dumb if they relate to the material being presented.

Stage 4: Out-of-Class Reworking

The notes you take in class are only one part of the effective study of lecture material. Out-of-class reworking of these notes is critical, and this is where the left-hand column of your note paper comes into use. Ideally, this reworking should be done immediately after the class ends, but this is not always possible. It must be done within 24 hours, however, to get full benefit from this strategy. Reworking class notes will not take more than 10 to 15 minutes to complete, but it will save you hours of study time later on.

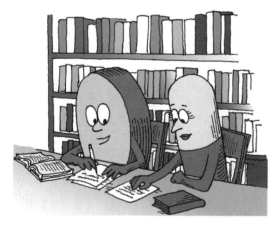

The following is the recommended method for reworking your class notes:

- **Read over the class notes**. Look for major topics, key ideas, terms, and the organization pattern. At this point you are not trying to remember everything you got from the lecture. You are looking for places where your notes are incomplete or confusing. If you read your notes soon after the lecture, you will be able to clarify points or add missing material because most of

what was said will still be fresh in your mind. If you wait until the next day (or worse, the next week), what is now only confusing will by then be a complete mystery. Taking the time to read your notes over soon after you take them will save much time and frustration later on.

- **Write topic heads for lecture segments** in the empty left-hand column of your notes. As you read your notes, identify the major topics that were discussed. For example, look at Chapter 12 in the text. The chapter title tells you that it is about general and local anaesthetics, but the information does not stop there. Further topics are discussed and divided into subgroups. Headings are necessary to break down very complex material into understandable blocks. You should be doing the same thing with your notes. Limit your labels to three to five words. You are not trying to rewrite class notes but to make the organization of the ideas crystal clear. Sometimes the notes on the chalkboard or Power Point slide will provide the labels for you. Sometimes the labels will be included in a lesson outline furnished by the instructor. Often, however, you will have to compose your own labels. With practice you will develop this skill. Keep at it. These labels are an essential aspect of the final stage of this note-taking method.

- **List vocabulary.** The left-hand column is also a great place to put content-specific vocabulary. Look again at Chapter 12. Notice that there is a glossary of terms for that chapter. This is provided so that you can immediately begin to focus on the content-specific vocabulary you will have to master for that chapter. You can create your own personal glossary of the terms used in the lecture. As you read over your notes, each time you encounter terms from the text or new terms introduced in the lecture, note the word in the left-hand column. Doing this will help you learn the needed vocabulary.

- **Expand.** Often during a lecture, you will only have time to write fragments of information. These may be meaningful at the time you write them but can be confusing later. Therefore, as you read your notes, fill in those places where there may be such gaps; otherwise, what was a small problem will become a big one later on. It will not take long, and it will pay off. You may use the left-hand column or the lines that you left blank for adding such information.

Remember: The reworking must be done the same day as the lecture for it to be efficient and productive. The longer the interval between the lecture and this reworking, the greater the likelihood of forgetting. When you read notes the same day as the lecture, you will be able to recall almost everything said. The reworking process will only take 10 minutes or so to complete, but it will pay off in a significantly improved set of class notes. Of equal importance is the fact that the reworking process is preparation for the final, critical stage in the note-taking process.

Stage 5: Frequent, Active Review

Notes, no matter how good, need to be **studied early and often.** Learning and memory depend on rehearsal, or review, and this must be an active process. Rereading notes will improve your understanding and memory somewhat, but there is a technique you can use that will accomplish much more. This technique will help you to be an active learner and encourage frequent rehearsal. It is also efficient because it will only take you 10 to 15 minutes to completely review 2 or 3 days' worth of class notes.

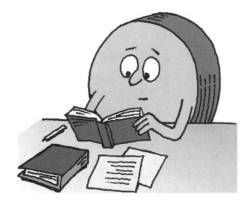

When to Review. The first review of your notes should be performed within 2 days of the lecture. If the lecture has taken place on Monday, your review should occur on Tuesday or Wednesday. Do not wait more than 2 days. Studies have repeatedly shown that we forget nearly 50% of what we learn in the first 24 hours after we learn it. The reworking process will slow the forgetting process, but it will not stop it. The longer you wait to review your notes, the more time it will take and the more difficult it will be when you finally do it.

When to do a second, third, or any additional reviews depends on the success of the previous review. Review each day until you find that you remember and understand 80% or more of the material (you have to be the judge). When this is accomplished, the next review can wait for 3 or 4 days. If you find that after the first review you recall or understand only 70% of the material (an average amount), then the next review should occur within 2 or 3 days. If the amount you remember is less than 70%, you should review the material the next day. You must assess your own performance on each review to determine how soon to schedule another

review. There are no hard and fast rules for this. A good review does not mean you have mastered the material forever, and what you remember clearly at one review may be the very thing you forget the next time around. **The only rule is to review frequently.** By doing this you will be well prepared for quizzes, tests, or any other measure of your learning.

How to Review. To review your notes, **cover the right-hand column** (class notes) with a blank sheet of paper. Look at the topics, vocabulary, and further notes that you added to the left-hand column during the reworking process. These will serve as your study guide for review. Look at the first topic heading you have written. It might be something like "Hypnotics." Turn that heading into one or more questions. What are hypnotics? When are they used? What are the side effects? Are there persons for whom hypnotics are inappropriate? Ask these questions aloud; do not just think them. **Framing questions orally is what makes this review active.** Now that you have asked a question, the next step is obvious. Answer it without looking at the covered notes. Say the answer aloud. This oral question-and-answer process forces you to state the information in your own words and style. In addition, you are relying on more faculties in your learning than just the visual one of rereading. You are speaking and listening, which is more active than just looking at the words. **Recall is strongly enhanced when you express the information in your own words.**

Another benefit of this review process is that it **helps identify what you do not know.** If you ask a question and find yourself struggling to respond, then it will be clear that this is something you have not yet mastered. When this happens, uncover the class notes pertaining to that topic and read what is needed. Sometimes only three or four words will be needed to trigger recall. When this happens, immediately cover the notes and resume your oral response. Sometimes you will have to read a large portion of the notes to trigger your memory. The reading is now focused on material that you have clearly identified as unknown. This means that your review time will be much more productive. Instead of reading everything known and unknown, you will now be concentrating on reinforcing the known material and studying the unknown. **The best way to prepare for a test is to take a test.** By using the question-and-answer model, you are creating and taking your own test. You may discover that many of the questions you asked yourself also appear in some form on the classroom test covering that same material. If you have already answered the question several times for yourself, it will be easy to answer it on the test.

Two-Page Split-Note Variation. There is a variation of the split-page note paper format that some students find works better for them. If you find that the 15-cm-wide right-hand column is too narrow for taking class notes, simply take your class notes on the right-hand page in your notebook and use the left-hand page for the reworking process. This allows more room for the charts, diagrams, or complex formulas that are often part of the lecture material in courses such as pharmacology. This two-page method will also allow you to incorporate text notes. To do this, divide the left-hand page into two columns of equal width. Use the right-hand column for the reworking of class notes and the left-hand column for text notes on the same topic.

On-the-Run Action. Record the information you find to be most difficult to remember on 3″ × 5″ cards and carry them with you in your pocket or purse. When you are waiting in traffic or for an appointment, just pull out the cards and review again. This "found" time may add points lost in the past to your test scores.

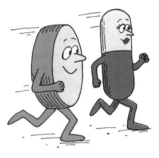

CHOOSE TO MASTER YOUR TEXTBOOKS

Many students find themselves falling asleep while reading their textbooks. Text material can be long, complex, sometimes confusing, and often highly technical. It can seem as though the more you read, the more there is to learn and the less you understand. Close the book and everything you have just read evaporates from your memory. If you feel like this, just remember—you are not alone. Every student feels this way. However, there are effective ways to maximize your learning and maybe even reduce the time it takes to do this.

Many different study systems have been devised to aid in the mastery of textbook material, and each has worked for some students. The model presented here is a combination of the best elements of this multitude of systems and is the best one for dealing with the subject matter in this pharmacology text.

Getting the most from a lecture requires active listening. The same active process applies to the reading of a textbook. Several techniques promote active reading. A good study system such as the PURR method presented in this textbook is one part of the process, but a good study system can be enhanced by reading with a pencil. Making text notations will help you concentrate and also make future review of the material more productive.

There are three notation systems:
- Highlighting-underlining
- Marginal notation
- Written text notes

Each of these notation systems has certain advantages and disadvantages. No single method will work perfectly all the time. Just as you must use different techniques to meet the different needs of your patients, you also need to use different techniques of text notation to meet the different needs you have as a learner. First, though, let's discuss two general guidelines that apply to the different systems of text notation.

General Guidelines

1. **Read first.** Before you begin to make any text notations, you must first read the material. The objective of text notations is to identify the important ideas, facts, and terms, just as this is the objective of listening during a lecture. If you attempt to mark text while reading it for the first time, everything will seem important and you will find yourself making far too many notations or highlighting far too much material.

2. **Be selective.** Be highly selective. The objective of text notation is much like that of taking notes during a lecture—to pick out the important ideas for immediate learning and for future review. If you have ever looked at a used textbook, you are sure to have seen that the previous owner has highlighted nearly every line on some pages. Excessive marking means the reader was not discerning the important ideas as he or she was reading. If you are taking separate handwritten notes, you should **limit what you write down** to the major headings and subheadings, important and unfamiliar vocabulary, and no more than two sentences of personal notes for each paragraph. The object is not to rewrite the chapter but to distill the important information. If you are highlighting, limit the material marked to no more than 20% to 25% of the total material. This is not to say that you must impose this limit on every paragraph, but it should be an overall goal.

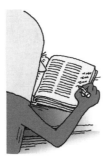

Text Notation Systems
Text Conventions

As you read and prepare for making text notations, be aware of certain conventions used throughout the text. These help the reader focus on what the authors consider important. By now you have noticed the use of headings in this study tips chapter. Look back at some of them and you will also notice that they are styled differently—some are all capitals; others have only the first letter of each word capitalized. These represent main topics and subtopics. Now look at a chapter in your text. Examine the way headings and bold facing draw your eyes to certain words, phrases, and portions of the page. These are text conventions provided by the authors to help you understand the organization of the material and the relationships within the text content. Other text conventions that you should note are numbered lists, bulleted lists, special display material, and the like.

Language Conventions

Another important aspect of text notation is to become language sensitive. In a class lecture, when you hear a professor say, for instance, "One of the most important first-generation anaesthetics was…," the words *most important* are a direct cue that this is a significant point for your notes. The same type of cueing often occurs in the text. The authors want to make certain that their important ideas are communicated to you, the reader. Because the authors cannot speak to you face to face, however, they must rely on a certain written style to get important points across. This means that you must become aware of that style so that you can identify these important ideas. For example, in a sentence saying "Opioids can be classified into four main categories," the phrase *four main categories* is the author's way of telling you not only what is coming but also what you should be taking note of.

Pay attention if a paragraph begins with the phrase "The most significant effects…." Whenever an author uses words or phrases such as these, it tells you that something important is being discussed. When you highlight text, phrases such as *most important, four main categories,* and *most significant* are the cues you should look for to help identify the most important information. The combination of text conventions and language conventions helps make the reading and marking of text more successful.

How to Highlight and Underline

Text marking is done to help in future review. This means that text marking is a personal process and should be used to point out only the most important information. The previous two sections on conventions gave you some concrete ideas on what to mark in your textbook. The main point is **read before you mark.**

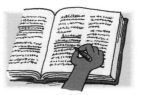

It is essential that you read meaningful blocks of text before you do any marking. A meaningful block may be as little as a single paragraph but never less. It may be as much as an entire chapter. In a text such as *Pharmacology for Canadian Health Care Practice*, in which the material is highly technical and challenging, it is unlikely that you will want to read more than a section of the chapter at a time before going back to highlight.

Look at Chapter 13. The first paragraph mentions the boldfaced terms *sedatives* and *hypnotics*. As you read this paragraph the first time, do not mark anything. Instead **read for a general understanding of the content**. After this, go back to the beginning of the section and note the following language conventions: *two basic elements, different stages, summarized, is known as,* and *four distinct stages*. These are all words and phrases that point out important information that should be highlighted. You may not actually need to highlight all the information flagged by these words and phrases. Some of it is probably already familiar to you because of earlier courses you have taken or earlier chapters you have read in this text. Avoid highlighting information you have already mastered.

Review
When

How soon after you have done some form of text notation should you review what you have highlighted? Ideally review should begin within 24 to 48 hours after the initial learning has occurred. Psychologists have studied learning, memory, and forgetting and have found that we forget approximately 50% of what we learn after the first day or two. Therefore, the sooner you begin to review, the easier it is to move learning from short-term memory (quickly learned and quickly forgotten) to long-term memory.

How

The process for reviewing any text notations follows the same general principles that apply to lecture notes. The intent is to make your review an active process in which real learning takes place. For example, if you have written questions in the text's margins, try to answer these questions without rereading the text. If you are able to answer the question to your satisfaction, then move on to the next question. If you have highlighted terms and definitions, cover the definition and try to define the term without looking at the text. If you are able to do this, you have effectively moved material into long-term memory. If you cannot define the term, then read the text definition. As you read, think about the meaning and think about strategies you might use to help you remember the term and definition the next time. You will find additional memory strategies in the later section on studying for exams. The key is always to focus on being an active learner.

How Often

How often you review is a personal matter. The best way to judge is to be aware of your success, or lack of it, in the current review session. If you do very well at recalling information, then you can probably wait 3 to 4 days for the next review. If the review goes okay, then the next session should take place within 2 days. If you find yourself reviewing your own notations with little understanding and limited memory, then the next review should take place the following day. Each time you review, it will get easier and faster, and as you practice this approach to reviewing your text notations, you will gradually acquire a good sense of how often you need to review to maintain mastery of the material.

CHOOSE TO PASS EXAMS

You can pass your exams by **applying the recommendations and strategies** offered in this section. Start by following the dozen basic rules of exam success.

Rules for Success on Exams

1. Accept your anxiety as normal. Tests are important, both in the short term, from the standpoint of grades and successful completion of this course, and also in the long term, from the standpoint of completing the program and getting your degree and eventually the job you want. This fact can cause stress.

2. Reduce your stress by **studying often, not long**. The most important rule in preparing for exams is simple—spend at least 15 minutes every day (Saturdays, Sundays, and holidays included) in reviewing the "old" material. The more time you can find for this each day, the better, but spend at least 15 minutes. This one action will do more to reduce test anxiety than anything else you do. The more time you devote to reviewing past material learned, the more confident you will feel about your knowledge of the topic. This confidence will accompany you into the classroom on the exam day, and it will help you get the test score that you want and are capable of. Just remember—**start the review process on the first day of the semester** and do some review every single day until the final exam.

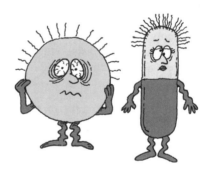

3. Balance your review time between your lecture notes, textbook notes or highlighting, and any handouts you may have been given.

4. Ask your instructor about the exam. If he or she says the test is mostly on the lecture, then you may want to spend more time reviewing your class notes. Ask about the type of questions that will be on the exam. Will the test consist entirely of multiple-choice questions? Will it have true-or-false items? Will there be matching, short-answer, or essay questions? You should not study any differently for a multiple-choice exam than you should for a short-answer or essay exam. However, knowing the type or types of questions that will be on the test will help you develop a strategy for quizzing yourself.

5. Work with your study group to create practice tests. For example, if you know the test will consist of multiple-choice questions, then as

you do your review, think of the kinds of questions you would ask if you were composing the test. Consider what would be a good question, what would be the right answer, and what would be other answers that would appear right but would in fact be incorrect.

6. Take the practice tests in each chapter and on the Evolve Web site (**http://evolve.elsevier.com/Canada/Lilley/pharmacology/**). Practice writing out the answers of short-answer or essay questions. **The best way to prepare for a test is to take one.**

7. **Study wisely, not hard.** Use the study strategies offered in this guide so you can save time and be able to get a good night's sleep the night before your exam. Cramming is not smart, and it is hard work that increases stress while reducing learning. When you cram, your mind is more likely to go blank during a test. When you cram, the information is in your short-term memory so you will need to relearn it before a comprehensive exam. Relearning takes more time. The stress caused by cramming may interfere with your sleep. Your brain needs sleep to function at its best.

8. Prepare for exams when and where you are most alert and able to concentrate. Use your personal prime time, which was discussed earlier in the time management section. If you are most alert at night, study at night. If you are most alert at 2 A.M., study in the early morning hours. Study where you can focus your attention and avoid distractions. This may be in the library or in a quiet corner of your home. The key point is to keep on doing what is working for you. If you are distracted or falling asleep, you may want to change when and where you are studying.

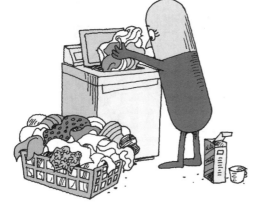

9. **Relax the last hour before an exam.** Your brain needs some recovery time to function effectively.

10. Survey the test before you start answering the questions. Plan how to complete the exam in the time allowed. Read the directions carefully and answer the questions you know for sure first.

11. Before turning in the exam, make sure that you have answered all of the questions. If you are to fill in the boxes on an answer sheet that will be read electronically, be sure you have put only one answer per line and that you have answered each question. If you must make a correction, be sure to erase carefully and thoroughly.

12. Celebrate your success. Congratulate yourself for choosing to pass your exam by applying the exam preparation and exam-taking skills that have been proven to work.

Strategies for Reviewing Class Notes

Look at your class notes. If you have been using the split-page model described earlier, you have made your own topic headings in the left-hand column beside the class notes. Cover the class notes and turn each heading into one or more questions. Think carefully about the answers and then answer aloud. By answering questions aloud, you are forcing yourself to think about what you know and organizing that knowledge in the way that is most meaningful to you. If you can answer your questions, then you have demonstrated that you know the material, and there is no immediate need to reread that section of notes. If you cannot answer one of your questions, then you know you need to review that material more intensively. Uncover the notes and read the pertinent ones. You are now using your review time effectively, because instead of just rereading everything, which invites boredom—or, worse yet, daydreaming—the rereading is directed at the material of which you are unsure. The result is more efficient use of your time and more effective learning.

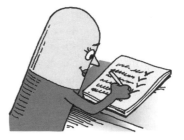

Strategies for Reviewing the Textbook

The technique you used for studying your class notes will also work for studying text material. As mentioned, in this book the authors have provided you with a variety of features that can help enormously. First, look at the objectives at the beginning of each chapter to be studied. Even if you have been assigned only small portions of the chapter, it is important to consider the objectives for the chapter as a whole. Ask yourself whether you have met these objectives. This is a quick way of assessing how much review may be necessary. If you feel confident that you have accomplished most of the objectives, then the review should go quickly. If you feel uncertain about many of them, then the review is going to take more time.

The next task is to consider the topic headings and language conventions. Use them in the same way as you have used the labels in your notes. Turn them into questions and answer these questions aloud. If you can answer them, then there is no need to reread. If you cannot, then you will need to reread the pertinent text.

Again, this way of reviewing is focusing your time and energy mostly where it is needed—on the material you have not yet mastered. Each time you review the text (or class notes), the sections of material you reread may differ. This is to be expected. You cannot remember everything forever, but if you spend time each day doing this type of review, you will remember more and for longer periods of time.

Strategies for Reviewing Terminology

One aspect of nursing that can seem overwhelming is the terminology. It is highly technical and specialized. Learning it poses the same kind of challenge as learning a foreign language. In fact, it almost is a foreign language. However, for the concepts and ideas to be mastered, the terms must be mastered. One of the best ways to go about doing this is to use a technique you probably learned in grade school—flash cards. Put each term on one side of a 3″ × 5″ note card and the definition or other essential information about the term on the back. Group together cards containing terms that have common word elements (e.g., terms beginning with *cardio*) or that concern common concepts (e.g., terms to do with renal function). The more relationships you can establish between words, the easier it will be to learn and remember them.

On-the-Run Action

Get in the habit of carrying a deck of 10 to 15 of these cards with you. When you have a few minutes, review as many cards as time allows. Some times start with the term side of the card and try to recall what is written on the back. Other times look at the definition on the back of the card and try to recall the term. Do not focus exclusively on term-to-definition learning because you may be given definitions or some variation on the exam and be asked to provide the terms.

Exam Time

This is it. The culmination of all your work—lectures, notes, flash cards, textbook readings, and handouts. **It is time to relax**. Test anxiety interferes with test performance. If you have put to use the learning techniques described in this chapter, you are ready for the exam. You have mastered the material, and you can do well on the exam. If you continue to experience test anxiety in spite of preparing thoroughly for the exam, it might be a good idea to visit a professional counselor on your campus.

Avoid cramming and remain confident in the learning techniques you have chosen to apply. This can usually control normal nervousness. Besides these learning techniques, however, techniques are also available for dealing with the various types of exam questions, and these are discussed in this section. None of these strategies can guarantee a 10-point jump in your test score. Only the degree to which you have mastered the material can make that sort of difference. However, each of the strategies described in this section may help you answer one or two questions correctly that you might otherwise have missed. **These test-taking strategies are not intended to replace regular study** and mastery; however, they are intended to enhance your test performance. If you use these strategies, you will see a positive gain in your test performance.

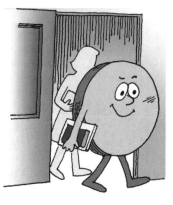

When the instructor passes out the exam, all your work and preparation are about to pay off, but do not just leap into the test. Take a couple of minutes to put yourself in a frame of mind for doing well on the test. At this point, you have a perfect test score—you have not answered any questions incorrectly yet. It is likely that you will get some answers wrong, but do not start out by making mistakes that cost you points that you should not have lost.

First, look over the entire test. Do not read it, but turn the pages and look at a question here and a question there. How many items are there on the test? Are all the questions of one type, or is there a mixture of types? Knowing in advance the length of the test and the types of questions helps you plan your strategy for taking the test.

Second, read the directions. This is the first opportunity you have to make a mistake that could cost points. Some directions for true-or-false questions may ask you to correct the statement and make it true. Others may ask you to justify your answer. When you respond with just a T or an F, you have lost important points because you did not read the directions.

Third, create a plan to complete the test in the time allowed. For example, if the test has 50 multiple-choice questions and the time limit is 40 minutes, then you know you will have to average a little better than one item per minute. Obviously you will need to allocate more time to essay questions if they are on the exam. Plan to glance at your watch or the classroom clock occasionally during the exam to make sure you are not losing time or going too quickly. Pace yourself. If you are answering questions quickly and are confident that the answers are right, do not worry about being ahead of schedule. If you spend too much time on individual questions, you may try to decide the answers to the last questions quickly, and this increases your chances of making errors. Planning a strategy for finishing the test within the time allowed helps you maintain a sharp focus on the task and enables you to do the best job possible.

Fourth, start answering the questions. If the test consists of only one type of question, then start with the first question. However, if the test has multiple-choice, true-or-false, and short-essay questions, for example, you must decide where it is best for you to start. If you find essay questions easy to do, then perhaps you should start with these. There is no reason you have to begin with the multiple-choice questions. On the other hand, if you find essay questions a challenge, then do not start with them. Begin the test in a way that will give you confidence.

Tips for Answering the Questions

- Start with the first question or with those types of questions you feel most confident answering. Wherever you choose to start, there

is a strategy you can use that can improve your test performance.

- Read the question carefully, and if you know the answer, indicate it and move on to the next question. If you cannot immediately think of the answer, give it a few seconds of thought. If the answer comes, indicate it and move on. If the answer still does not come or if the question is confusing, then skip to the next question.

- In the first pass through the exam, answer what you know and skip what you do not know. Answering the questions you are sure of increases your confidence and saves time. This is buying you time to devote to the questions with which you have more difficulty.

- Notice that the subjects of the questions on a particular exam are related, that the answers to questions you have skipped may be provided by other questions on the test, or that a later question may trigger recall of the correct answer. Skipping questions you are unsure of offers one more opportunity to get the correct answer.

- After you have gone through the entire test completing the questions that you are confident you can correctly answer, go back to the items you skipped. First check the time, however, so you know how much time you have left to answer these questions. On this second pass through the exam, you will often be surprised at how many questions you now can answer that drew a complete blank before.

- Answer every question. A question without an answer is the same as a wrong answer. *Go ahead and guess.* You have studied for the test and you know the material well. You are not making a random guess based on no information. You are guessing based on what you have learned and your best assessment of the question.

- When you have answered all the questions on a page, put a check in the upper right corner of this page. Avoid going back and second guessing yourself. There is nothing worse than changing right answers to wrong ones. Have confidence in your own knowledge and let go of the test. If you are the first person to complete a test and are sure of what you did, then turn it in. At the same time, do not let what others in the class are doing affect your test strategy. If you are the last person to turn the test in, it does not mean you know less than those who were faster. It simply means that you are a careful, thoughtful test taker.

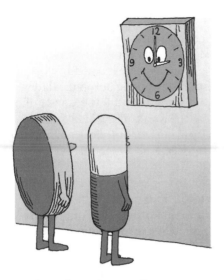

Strategies for Specific Types of Questions

For each type of question there are particular strategies you can use that can help prevent incorrect responses. Many times students miss questions not because of a lack of information but because of a poor strategy. Sometimes the error stems from misreading a question, for instance, overlooking a key word such as *not*, or from choosing an answer that does not quite fit the question asked. Errors like these can be costly. Expect to find some questions on a test to which you do not remember the answer or that are worded in a confusing way. A perfect test score is a great goal, but be realistic and accept the fact that perfect scores may be few and far between. At the same time, do not lose points because of careless and preventable errors.

Strategy for Multiple-Choice Questions

Multiple-choice questions can be challenging, because students think that they will recognize the right answer when they see it or that the right answer will somehow stand out from the other choices. This is a dangerous misconception. The more carefully the question is constructed, the more each of the

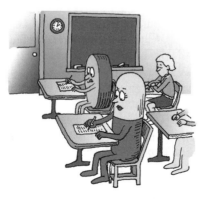

choices will seem like the correct response. The successful student can do several things to improve performance on multiple-choice questions.

Before the strategies for analyzing multiple-choice questions are discussed, it is important to understand each part of a question and its purpose. There are three parts to a multiple-choice question: stem, distractors, and the correct choice.

First, there is the **question stem**. This is the complete question that one, or more, of the response choices will answer.

EXAMPLE:

If excessive amounts of water-soluble vitamins are ingested, what usually happens?

Notice that this could just as easily be a short-answer question. In this case, the stem is a complete sentence that should be answered by one of the response choices. The stem can also be an incomplete statement that one or more of the response choices completes correctly.

EXAMPLE:

The likelihood that a drug will have therapeutic effects increases dramatically when

This statement is incomplete, and you must pick out the response choice that best completes it.

The second part of multiple-choice questions is the **distractors**. These are the response choices that do not best answer or complete the stem. They are known as distractors because that is their purpose, to distract you from the best choice. Good distractors are usually very similar to the **best choice**. If you have not studied enough, a good distractor will be a very tempting choice, but you must reduce the allure of distractors.

The third and final part of all multiple-choice questions is the best choice. This is the choice you want to pick. Notice that it is the "best" choice. In many multiple-choice questions there may be more than one response choice that appears to answer the stem, and the differences between the responses may be slight. Your task is therefore to identify the option that best answers the stem, not necessarily the only right choice.

Recall. The most reliable way to ensure that you select the correct response to a multiple-choice question is to recall it. Depend on your learning and memory to furnish the answer to the question. To do this, read the stem, and then *stop!* Do not look at the response options yet. Try to recall what you know and, based on this, what you would give as the answer. After you have taken a few seconds to do this, look at all of the choices and select the one that most nearly matches the answer you recalled. It is important that you consider all the choices and not just choose the first option that seems to fit the answer you recall. Remember the distractors. Choice B may look okay, but choice D may be worded in a way that makes D a slightly better choice. If you do not weigh all the choices, you are not maximizing your chances of correctly answering each question.

Once you have decided on an answer, there is one more important step before you mark it. Look at the stem again. Does your choice answer the question that was asked? If the question stem asks "why," be sure the response you have chosen is a reason. If the question stem is singular, then be sure the option is singular, and the same for plural stems and plural responses. Many times, checking to make sure that the choice makes sense in relation to the stem will reveal the correct answer.

This is the most reliable technique to use for answering multiple-choice questions. If you do this for every multiple-choice question on the test, your accuracy rate will be very high, and you will not need any further strategy. Unfortunately, however, recall does not always work, and when it does not, there are some additional strategies you can apply to improve your chances of picking the correct answer.

Recognition and Elimination. Read each of the answer options carefully. Usually at least one of them will be clearly wrong. Eliminate this one from consideration. Now you have reduced the number of response choices by one and improved the odds. Continue to analyze the options. If you can eliminate one more choice in a four-option question, you have reduced the odds to 50/50, the same as the odds of correct random guessing for true-or-false questions. There are still some strategies that will help you pick the best choice. In addition, while you are eliminating the wrong choices, recall often occurs. One of the options may serve as a trigger that causes you to remember what a few seconds ago had seemed completely forgotten.

LOOK-ALIKE ANSWERS. After you have eliminated one or more choices, you may discover that two of the options are very similar. This can be very helpful, because it may mean that one of these look-alike answers is the best choice and the other is a very good distractor. Test both of these options against the stem. Ask yourself which one completes the incomplete statement grammatically and which one answers the question more fully and completely. The option that best completes or answers the stem is the one you should choose. Here, too, pause for a few seconds, give your brain time to reflect, and recall may occur.

ABSOLUTES. The presence of absolute words and phrases can also help you determine the correct answer to a multiple-choice item. If an answer choice contains an absolute (e.g., *none, never, must, cannot*), be very cautious. Remember that there are not many things in this world that are absolute, and in an area as complex as pharmacology, an absolute in an option may be reason to eliminate it from consideration as the best choice. This is only a guideline and should not be taken to be true 100% of the time; however, it can help you reduce the number of choices.

NEGATIVES AND EXCEPTIONS. In the stem "A drug reaction could include all but which of these symptoms?" the phrase *all but* tells you to choose the response that is an exception. *All but one* of the choice options is a symptom. In this case, the option that is not a symptom is the best choice. If you look at the options and see several that seem correct, look at the stem again. It may be that you have overlooked an exception phrase such as *all but* or *all but one*. A similar stem wording that can throw you off is a negative or negative prefix. The stem "It is generally *not* a good idea to administer adult dosages to..." is asking you to select the answer that names the inappropriate, not appropriate, recipient of a medication. The word *not* helps identify the answer.

All these strategies can help you analyze the response choices so that you have the best possible chance of selecting the correct choice. When you are ready to mark the answer, keep in mind that the final step is always to test your response against the stem.

If, after you have tried all of these strategies, you find yourself still unable to choose a response, there is one final strategy. Ask the instructor for clarification of the question. There is nothing to lose by asking and everything to gain. The worst that can happen is that the instructor will tell you that he or she cannot answer your question. The best that can happen is that the instructor will rephrase the question in a way that resolves the problem for you.

When asking for such clarification, try to phrase your question in a way that encourages a response. Do not simply state that you do not understand the question. This is generally not the approach that invites an answer. If you are having trouble with a term in the stem or response choices, ask for a definition. If there is a phrase that is unclear or a response choice that is confusing, ask for clarification. Anything you do to make your question more specific increases the likelihood that the instructor will answer it.

After all other avenues have been exhausted, remember the final rule. **Never leave a question unanswered.** Even if answering is no more than an educated guess on your part, go ahead and mark an answer. You might be right, but if you leave it blank, you will certainly be wrong and lose precious points.

Strategy for Short-Answer and Essay Questions

Notice that this strategy applies to both short-answer and essay questions. Both types of questions require careful thought and planning before you write an answer. It is helpful to get into the habit of regarding short-answer questions as short-essay questions. Too often students lose points on short-answer questions by being too brief. A short answer should usually consist of three or four sentences, but frequently students interpret "short answer" to mean four or five words.

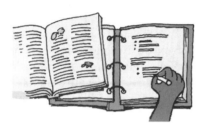

Start answering these questions by analyzing the question carefully and then framing a response that will fully answer it. Assume that the reader—in this case, the course instructor—does not know anything and that you have to explain it all. Short-answer and essay questions require you to show what you know. Do not assume that the instructor can read your mind or read between the lines of your response to discern what you knew but did not include. It is better to have a little more than was needed in your answer than not enough. Extra information will not hurt, but missing information will always cost points. Once again, remember that the idea is to gain a point here and there throughout the test, which will result in a higher score and a better grade for the course.

Two Key Issues

1. In writing answers to short-answer and essay questions, it is essential to answer exactly the question that is asked. This means that you must understand the question before you do any writing. Unlike with true-or-false and multiple-choice questions, which you should try to answer using every possible strategy before seeking help, with these questions you should ask for help before doing anything. The first opportunity you have to lose points in an essay question occurs with the first reading of the question. If you misread the question, you may write an excellent answer but not the right one. Such a mistake can be costly.
2. A good answer must be organized so that it is clear and logical to the reader. Do not read a question and start writing down whatever ideas spring to mind. Spend a minute or two thinking and planning the structure of the answer so that your ideas are clearly stated and the supporting details relate directly to each idea. Your instructor, the reader, will have a difficult time grading your essay if he or she has to read it two or three times to figure out what you were trying to say. Organization and clarity of expression really pay off in essay exams.

Five Steps to Good Essay Answers

1. **Read the questions carefully.** As was discussed earlier, misreading the question can result in a high-quality answer that does not address the question asked. Read and think about the question's major focus. Do not jump on the first familiar phrase or term and start writing without further thought.

2. **Decide on an approach.** Telling you to read the question carefully is good advice, but without some strategy to apply to the reading it might be difficult advice to carry out. Here is a strategy to help you read carefully and begin to plan your answer. Look at the question as you read, and identify the words and phrases that tell you what to do. Some standard "what-to-do" words and phrases are used consistently in essay questions, such as *discuss, compare, contrast, explain, tell why,* and *analyze.* Circle each of these words or phrases as you read the question. The second part of the decision step is to underline what you are to write about. This circling and underlining will force a careful reading of the question and help you begin the process of organizing the answer. The sample question that follows is marked to show the circle and underline strategy.

SAMPLE QUESTION:

(Discuss) the _ways_ in which _child and older adult patients_ are _alike_ in _determining_ appropriate dosage. (Explain) _why adult dosage_ may be _inappropriate and_ the _dangers_ in _using adult dosage_ in these special populations.

3. **Compile a brief written outline.** Before you start writing your answer, take a few minutes to organize the points you want to cover. This should not be an elaborate outline with roman numerals, capital letters, and arabic numbers, but rather a quick sketch of the question and the points you want to make in the answer. The circle-and-underline step described earlier will help make this easy to do.

SAMPLE OUTLINE*:

Discuss
- Child and older adult patients' similarity with regard to drug dosage
    - Body weight factor
    - Organ function

Explain
- Reasons adult dosage inappropriate
    - Drugs not tested on pediatric and elderly population
- Dangers of adult dosage
    - Possible organ damage
    - Increased absorption and possible side effects

Sketching out an outline like this will organize your ideas, speed your writing, and ensure that you are answering the question asked.

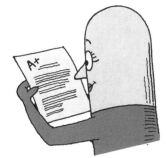

4. Write an answer. With the question analyzed and a quick outline in place, it is time to put your answer on paper. The basic structure of an exam essay or answer to a short-answer question is the same as that for an in-class composition on an assigned topic. Every rule on which composition teachers insist for writing assignments should be followed in writing essay answers.

Any answer of more than four or five sentences should follow the basic three-part essay structure of introduction, body, and conclusion.

The **introduction** should be only one or two sentences long. It tells the reader what you are going to present in your answer. There is a relatively simple way to write an essay introduction. State the question positively and add a few words that show the main points you intend to make in your answer.

SAMPLE INTRODUCTION:

Child and older adult patients have a number of similarities that must be considered in determining

drug dosage. Two of the most important are body weight and organ function, and these factors can make adult dosages inappropriate for these two populations.

These two sentences tell the reader exactly what you plan to discuss. From this point on, it becomes your task to explain why those two are important and how they affect drug dosage. You have told the reader what to expect, and you have begun to organize your answer.

The **body** is the most important part of any essay answer. In it you want to state the ideas, concepts, and points that you believe answer the question. These should be stated clearly and positively. Do not ramble on trying to cover all the possible variations that might fit into an answer. Decide on the most important, most significant points you have to make. Then state them and support and explain with relevant details that show how and why your points answer the question. For short-answer questions where three to five sentences are expected, drop the introduction and conclusion, and put all of your energy into a clear, concise body.

For the **conclusion**, there should be a concluding sentence or two to let the reader know that you have finished. Like the introduction, it should be brief and direct. Restate the question, and summarize the key points made in your answer.

SAMPLE CONCLUSION:

It is evident that older adult and child patients are very similar in their responses to drug dosages. Clearly the factors of body weight and organ function will play a major role in determining the appropriate dosages for these two groups.

5. Read the answer. The writing has been completed. Before you turn in the paper, take another minute or two and read over what you have written. Look for errors that would make the reader pause, question what you have said, or be unable to read a word or phrase. Sometimes the mind works much faster than the pen, and a word or phrase is left out in writing. Use a caret (^) and insert the word or phrase where it belongs. If your writing got a little sloppy and a word is hard to read, cross it out and print it clearly right above. Proofreading and correcting small errors like these will make the answer easier to read and understand. Anything that contributes to the overall quality of an answer will influence the grade in a positive manner. You will not have time to rewrite an answer, but you should correct obvious errors.

*This is a model of the process of the Decision and Outline steps. It is not to be viewed as an accurate outline of pharmacological content.

Strategy for True-or-False Questions

True-or-false items outwardly appear to be fairly simple. After all, the statement is either true or false. The odds of answering correctly are 50/50, and if all else fails, a coin toss can decide the issue. Appearances are deceiving, however, and true-or-false questions can be very challenging to answer. Good test strategy should be applied to answer all types of questions, because the object is to get the best score you can, and this represents the total points for all correct answers.

Read the Question. Reading the question may seem like such an obvious part of all test-taking strategies that it may appear absurd even to be told to do this. If you do not pay careful attention to the wording of true-or-false statements, however, you are increasing the odds of making an otherwise avoidable error. Take the time to read and understand the statement. Read it all the way through to the end. Do not jump to conclusions based on half the statement.

Assume That the Statement Is True. As you read each true-or-false statement, begin with the assumption that the statement is true. The idea behind this strategy is that it will cause you to read the statement carefully, which will result in your choosing the correct answer. This approach to reading the statement makes the reading an active process, because you are then reading to confirm the truth in the statement. You will be analyzing the statement as you read, looking for any information that would contradict or change the statement from true to false. You will also be choosing your answer as you read rather than waiting to the end to decide whether the statement was true or false. Obviously not every statement will be true, but this step makes you a much more thoughtful reader, and that encourages better test performance.

Remember one other important rule when analyzing true-or-false statements. **If any part of the statement is false, then the entire statement is false.** There may be only one altered word or prefix (such as un- or anti-) that changes a statement from true to false, but that is all that is required.

Strategies for Analysis. Sometimes, no matter how carefully you have read the question, the answer is not immediately obvious. When that happens, there are a number of strategies you can use to analyze the question. Using these strategies will not guarantee that you will get the correct answer, but they will often help you see something about the statement you might have overlooked and assist you in identifying the correct answer.

ABSOLUTES AND QUALIFIERS. Absolutes are words such as *none*, *never*, *all*, or *always*. These

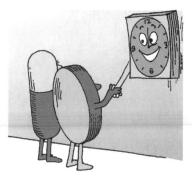

words mean that there are absolutely no exceptions to the statement. For instance, the statement "All birds fly" means just that. Every bird, past, present, and future, has flown or does fly. If there is or has been just one bird that has not flown or does not fly, then the statement is false. All in this statement is an absolute. True-or-false statements that contain such absolutes are usually false. In an area as complex as pharmacology, it is unlikely that there are many absolutes. If you are struggling with a question that has you stumped, look for absolute words. They may help you determine the answer.

On the other hand, there are words that suggest the possibility of exceptions. Such words or phrases are called qualifiers; examples of these are *some, possibly, in most cases,* and *will generally*. "Most birds can fly" is an example of a qualified statement. The word *most* tells you that some not precisely specified number of all birds can fly. This makes it more probable that the statement is true.

STATED IN THE NEGATIVE. A true-or-false statement that is rendered in the negative can be difficult to answer. To draw on the earlier example, "It is not true that all birds can fly" is such a statement. The word not in this statement can make it much more complex to read and answer. There is a relatively simple way to deal with this type of statement. Read it as though the negative were not included, so that it becomes "It is true that all birds can fly." This statement is clearly false. Because the word *not* reverses the meaning of the statement, this makes the statement "It is not true that all birds can fly" true. Simply put, if the statement is true without the negative, then it becomes false with the negative. Similarly, if it is false without the negative, then it is true with the negative.

STRINGS. A string is a true-or-false statement that requires careful attention. It is a statement that contains a list of several words or phrases, but often one or more of the words or phrases is false. It is easy to read the statement and see that the first two or three words or phrases are true but then overlook the one that is incorrect, with the consequence that you mark the answer as true when it is actually false. An example of a string is "First-generation cephalsporins, such as cefadroxil, cloxacillin, cefazolin, and cephalexin, are antibiotics specifically active against gram-negative bacteria." As you read this statement, it is easy to be lured by the words *such as* into thinking the statement is true without noting the fact that cloxacillin is in fact a penicillinase-resistant penicillin, not a cephalosporin. The statement is false, but the string can trick you into thinking the statement is true.

These strategies for analyzing true-or-false items can help you increase the number of correct answers, but they are not intended to replace study and learning. The best way to perform well on any test is to know the answers based on your own learning. When the answer does not immediately come to mind, however, apply these strategies. Although they will not necessarily lead to a 10-point difference in your score, they may help you add 2 points to your score. Better scores mean better course grades, and of course, this results in improved self-confidence and improved chances of success.

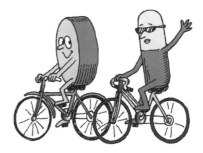

CONCLUSION

Remember: These study tips are only as valuable as you make them!

Chapter 1

Nursing Practice in Canada and Drug Therapy

CHAPTER REVIEW

Choose the best answer for each of the following.

1. Which phase of the nursing process requires the nurse to establish a comprehensive baseline of data concerning a particular patient?
   a. Assessment
   b. Planning
   c. Implementation
   d. Evaluation

2. The nurse may revise or eliminate unrealistic goals during which phase of the nursing process?
   a. Assessment
   b. Planning
   c. Implementation
   d. Evaluation

3. Prescribed medications are prepared and administered during which phase of the nursing process?
   a. Assessment
   b. Planning
   c. Implementation
   d. Evaluation

4. Which of the following must occur for a goal statement to be patient centred?
   a. Family input is essential.
   b. The patient must be involved in establishing the goal(s).
   c. The nurse must develop the goal(s).
   d. The physician must be involved in establishing the goal(s).

5. Which of the following is part of a complete medication history?
   a. Use of "street" drugs
   b. Current laboratory work
   c. Past history of surgeries
   d. Family history

6. The nurse prioritizes the nursing diagnoses during which phase of the nursing process?
   a. Assessment
   b. Planning
   c. Implementation
   d. Evaluation

Label each of the following as either objective data (O) or subjective data (S).

7. Below is a list of data gathered from an assessment of Ms. Biehle, a young woman visiting the clinic with what she describes as "maybe an ulcer."

   _____ Ms. Biehle says that she smokes a pack of cigarettes a day.

   _____ She is 165 cm tall and weighs 61.2 kg.

   _____ The nurse finds that her pulse rate is 68 beats per minute and her blood pressure is 128/72 mm Hg.

   _____ Her stool was tested for occult blood by a laboratory technician; the results were negative.

   _____ Ms. Biehle says that she does not experience nausea, but she reports pain and heartburn, especially after eating popcorn, something she and her husband have always done while watching TV before bedtime.

   _____ She experiences occasional increases in stomach pain, "a feeling of heat" in her abdomen and chest at night when she lies down, and increased incidents of heartburn.

CRITICAL THINKING AND APPLICATION

Answer the following questions on a separate sheet of paper.

8. Identify the "10 Rights" of drug administration, and specify ways to ensure that each of these rights is addressed.

9. The following items will help you review the nursing process.

   Data are collected during the (a.) _____ phase of the nursing process.

   Data can be classified as (b.) _____ or (c.) _____.

   To formulate the nursing diagnosis, the nurse must first (d.) _____ the information collected.

   The planning phase includes identification of (e.) _____ and (f.) _____.

   The (g.) _____ phase consists of initiation and completion of the nursing care plan.

   The (h.) _____ phase is ongoing and includes monitoring the patient's response to medication and determining the status of goals.

CASE STUDY

Read the scenario and answer the following questions on a separate sheet of paper.

A 69-year-old woman has been admitted because of nausea and vomiting. She also has a diagnosis of hepatitis C. She says she stopped drinking 3 years ago but has had increasing problems with peripheral edema and shortness of breath and has had trouble getting out of bed or chairs independently. Laboratory results show elevated liver enzyme studies, and decreased sodium and potassium levels. Her blood pressure is 160/98 mm Hg, her pulse rate is 98 beats/min, and her respiratory rate is 24 breaths/min. She is afebrile and states that she is having slight abdominal pain.

1. From the brief facts given, what information will be important to consider when obtaining a drug history?

2. The physician wrote the following drug order:

May 4, 2010
Give furosemide now.
              Charles Simmons, MD

Patient's Name: Jane Doe	F	Age: 69
Medical Record No: 1234567		DOB: 16/1/41

   What elements, if any, are missing from the above medication order? What should the nurse do next?

3. After the order is clarified, the pharmacy sends up furosemide (Lasix) 80 mg tablets, but the patient is unable to swallow them because of her nausea. A colleague suggests giving the furosemide to her as an intravenous injection. What should the nurse do next?

4. After the patient has received the dose of furosemide, what should the nurse do?

Chapter 2

Pharmacological Principles

CHAPTER REVIEW

Provide the best answer for each of the following.

1. Number the following drug forms in order of speed of dissolution and absorption, with 1 being the fastest and 4 being the slowest:

   a. _____ Capsules

   b. _____ Enteric-coated tablets

   c. _____ Elixirs

   d. _____ Powders

2. When considering the various routes of drug elimination, the nurse is aware that elimination occurs mainly from which of the following?
   a. Kidney tubules and skin
   b. Skin and lungs
   c. Bowel and kidney tubules
   d. Lungs and gastrointestinal tract

3. The nurse is aware that excessive dosages, poor circulation, faulty metabolism, or inadequate excretion may result in which drug effect?
   a. Tolerance
   b. Cumulative effect
   c. Incompatibility
   d. Antagonistic effect

4. The nurse knows that drug half-life is the amount of time required for 50% of a drug to do which of the following?
   a. Be absorbed by the body
   b. Reach a therapeutic level
   c. Exert a response
   d. Be eliminated by the body

5. The nurse recognizes that drugs given by which route will be altered by the first-pass effect?
   a. Oral
   b. Sublingual
   c. Subcutaneous
   d. Intravenous

6. If a drug binds with an enzyme and thereby prevents the enzyme from binding to its normal target cell, it will produce an effect known as which of the following?
   a. Receptor interaction
   b. Enzyme stimulation
   c. Enzyme interaction
   d. Nonspecific interaction

Match each field of study with its corresponding "job" description.

7. _____ Pharmaceutics

8. _____ Pharmacokinetics

9. _____ Pharmacodynamics

10. _____ Pharmacogenetics

11. _____ Pharmacotherapeutics

12. _____ Pharmacognosy

a. Lisa is researching botanical and zoological sources of drugs to treat multiple sclerosis. She is part of a university research team that is currently experimenting with varying the biochemical composition and therapeutic effects of several possible new drugs.

b. Vladimir works for a pharmaceutical corporation. One of its new drugs looks promising, and Vladimir's company is experimenting

13. _____ Toxicology

14. _____ Teratogenesis

15. _____ Prophylactic therapy

with dose forms for this investigational new drug. He is responsible for measuring the relationship between the physiochemical properties of the dosage form and the clinical therapeutic response.

c. Meiko examines case studies of patients with similar conditions and drug therapies to determine similarities based on clinical observations.

d. Hamische researches various poisons and studies and is particularly concerned with the detection and treatment of the effects of drugs and chemicals in certain mammals.

e. Steven represents a research firm that subcontracts with Health Canada to observe and report on drug-induced congenital anomalies and the toxic effects drugs can have on the developing fetus.

f. Nirmala and Phil have spent the last 3 years gathering family histories, legal case reports, and current clinical data to identify possible genetic factors that influence individuals' responses to meperidine (Demerol) and related drugs.

g. Amjad works on a study that is gathering data on the use of two different drugs for the treatment of rheumatoid arthritis.

h. Jin Hee's laboratory monitors drug distribution rates between various body components, from absorption through excretion. Recently, her laboratory was able to suggest a positive change in the dosage regimen of an injectable drug, bringing her firm a prestigious award.

i. Gregory's research unit recently recommended two new contraindications for the use of a newly marketed drug after discovering previously unknown biochemical and physiological interactions of this drug with another unrelated drug.

CRITICAL THINKING AND APPLICATION

Answer the following questions on a separate sheet of paper.

16. Mr. Zhang enters the trauma centre in some distress. He is experiencing symptoms that demand quick absorption of a drug. If presented with the following choices, which route of administration would the nurse use: subcutaneous or intramuscular? Mr. Zhang's physician asks the nurse to further increase absorption, mechanically. How can the nurse do this?

17. Ms. Clark has had ovarian cancer for over a year. She is now in the late stages of her illness and in severe pain. She has been admitted to a hospice unit and is receiving morphine through a patient-controlled analgesia pump. This is an example of which type of drug therapy: acute, maintenance, supplemental, or palliative? Explain your answer.

CASE STUDY

Read the scenario and answer the following questions on a separate sheet of paper.

A 65-year-old man with liver cirrhosis is admitted to the medical-surgical unit with nausea and vomiting. He also has a diagnosis of heart failure. The nurse notes that his serum albumin level is low. The physician has written admission orders, and the nurse is trying to make the patient comfortable. He is to take nothing by mouth except for clear liquids. An intravenous infusion of dextrose 5% in water at 50 mL/hr has been ordered, and the unit nurses have had difficulty inserting his intravenous line.

1. One of the drugs ordered is known to reach a maximum level in the body of 200 mg/L and has a half-life of 2 hours. If this maximum level of 200 mg/L is reached at 4 P.M., what will the drug's level in the body be at 10 P.M.?

2. Explain what factors from this patient's history would affect the following:

    a. Absorption

    b. Distribution

    c. Metabolism

    d. Excretion

3. Placement of a peripherally inserted central catheter (PICC) has been ordered. The physician writes an order for a dose of an intravenous antibiotic to be given before this procedure is carried out. What is the reason for this order?

4. This patient is also receiving digoxin (Lanoxin) for heart failure. This drug is known to have a low therapeutic index. Explain this concept.

Chapter 3

Considerations for Special Populations

CHAPTER REVIEW

Choose the best answer for each of the following.

1. Which physiological factor is most responsible for the differences in the pharmacokinetic and pharmacodynamic behaviour of drugs in neonates and adults?
   a. Infant's stature
   b. Infant's smaller weight
   c. Immaturity of neonatal organs
   d. Adult's longer exposure to toxins

2. When considering drug therapy in children, the nurse recognizes that which group of drugs is the most toxic for children?
   a. phenobarbital, morphine, and acetylsalicylic acid
   b. phenobarbital, morphine, and atropine
   c. theophylline, atropine, and digoxin
   d. morphine, atropine, and digoxin

3. Most drug references recommend that dosages for children be based on which of the following?
   a. Total body water content
   b. Fat-to-lean mass ratio
   c. Height as measured in centimetres
   d. Milligrams per kilogram of body weight

4. When considering drug dosages in older adults, the nurse recognizes that drug dosages in the older adult should be based on which of the following?
   a. More on age than on height or weight
   b. More on weight than on age
   c. On the total body water content
   d. On the glomerular filtration rate

5. When giving medications to the older adult, the nurse should keep in mind the changes that occur due to aging. Which of the following statements regarding changes in the older adult patient are true? Select all that apply.
   a. Total body water content is decreased as body composition changes.
   b. Gastric pH is less acidic because of reduced hydrochloric acid production.
   c. Protein albumin binding sites are increased because of decreased protein.
   d. Fat content is increased because of decreased lean body mass and altered total body water.
   e. The absorptive surface area of the gastrointestinal tract is increased due to flattening and blunting of the villi.

Match each U.S. FDA pregnancy safety category with its corresponding description.

6. _____ Category A

7. _____ Category B

8. _____ Category C

9. _____ Category D

10. _____ Category X

a. Possible fetal risk in humans is reported; however, the potential benefits may, in selected cases, outweigh the risks and warrant the use of these drugs in pregnant women.

b. Studies indicate no risk to animal fetuses; information in humans is not available.

c. Fetal abnormalities are reported, and positive evidence of fetal risk in humans is available from animal and/or human studies.

d. Studies indicate no risk to the fetus.

e. Adverse effects are reported in animal fetuses; information in humans is not available.

CRITICAL THINKING AND APPLICATION

Answer the following questions on a separate sheet of paper.

11. A nurse works at a community clinic frequented by a number of older adult patients. Mrs. Benerjee comes to the clinic complaining of dizziness and nausea. As the nurse takes her medication history, she shows him her "pill box." Inside, he sees almost a dozen different pills, all to be taken at noon. How could this happen? How could she possibly need so many medications at the same time?

12. The physician confirms that Mrs. Benerjee's "new symptoms," as she refers to them, are a result of polypharmacy. She protests, telling the nurse, "My dear, I've got news for the doctor. I've had to take lots of drugs at the same time all my life. It never bothered me before. Why would it now when I'm even more used to it?" Explain at least three physiological changes that occur with aging and how these changes affect pharmacokinetics and pharmacodynamics.

CASE STUDY

Read the scenario and answer the following questions on a separate sheet of paper.

The nurse is performing telephone triage in a pediatric clinic. A mother calls about her 28-month-old toddler, who has had chicken pox for 2 days. She wants to give acetylsalicylic acid (Aspirin) because the toddler's fever is 38.3°C, but is unsure because her toddler "hates to take pills."

1. Should the mother use acetylsalicylic acid for this fever? Check a drug reference, if needed, for developmental considerations in this situation.

2. The mother states that her husband is going to the drug store for some medicine. What would the nurse tell her about the dosage form of an antipyretic for her toddler?

3. When the husband returns from the store, he shows the mother the bottle of Children's Acetaminophen Suspension Cherry Flavour that was recommended by the store's pharmacist. He wonders, though, why the pharmacist would need to know the toddler's weight before suggesting this medication. Explain.

4. The toddler receives a dose of 5 mL per the directions according to his weight of 12.7 kg. Later, when his 5-year-old sister needs a dose, she receives 7.5 mL because of her weight of 20.4 kg. If the drug contains 160 mg per 5 mL, then how much medication did the 5-year-old receive in her dose?

5. What should the parents look for when evaluating the children's response to a dose of acetaminophen?

Chapter 4

Ethnocultural, Legal, and Ethical Considerations

CHAPTER REVIEW

Choose the best answer for each of the following.

1. What is the primary purpose of Health Canada's Therapeutic Products Directorate?
   a. To allow pharmaceutical companies a time frame of noncompetitiveness with generic drugs
   b. To ensure the safety, efficacy, and quality of drugs sold on the market
   c. To direct and monitor the clinical trials of therapeutic drugs
   d. To monitor the import and export of foods and drugs

2. Which of the following Health Canada regulations applies to the sale of probiotics, amino acids, and essential fatty acids?
   a. Natural Health Products Regulations
   b. Precursor Control Regulations
   c. Supplements and Dietary Products Regulations
   d. Benzodiazepines and Other Targeted Substances Regulations

3. What is the ethical principle of "do no harm" known as?
   a. Autonomy
   b. Beneficence
   c. Confidentiality
   d. Nonmaleficence

4. Which of the following is considered a phase in investigational drug studies? Select all that apply.
   a. Phase I: drug safety study
   b. Phase II: drug effectiveness study
   c. Phase IV: branded versus generic drugs comparison study
   d. Phase III: drug duration and long-term effects study

5. Which of the following is the correct definition for *placebo*?
   a. An investigational drug used in a new drug study
   b. An inert substance that is not a drug
   c. A legend drug that requires a prescription
   d. A substance that is not approved as a drug but is used as a natural health product

6. During an admission assessment, which of the following would be part of the findings of a cultural assessment?
   a. The patient uses acetylsalicytic acid as needed for pain.
   b. The patient has a history of hypertension.
   c. The patient is allergic to shellfish.
   d. The patient does not eat pork products for religious reasons.

Match each investigational drug study phase with its corresponding description.

7. _____ Phase I

8. _____ Phase II

9. _____ Phase III

10. _____ Phase IV

a. A study using small numbers of volunteers who have the disease or disorder that the drug is meant to diagnose or treat. Subjects are monitored for drug efficacy and adverse effects.

b. Postmarketing studies conducted by drug companies to obtain further proof of the drug's therapeutic effects.

c. A study that involves a large number of patients at research centres and is designed to monitor for infrequent adverse effects and identify any associated risks. Double-blind, placebo-controlled studies eliminate patient and researcher bias.

    d. A study that uses small numbers of healthy volunteers, as opposed to volunteers afflicted with the target ailment, to determine dosage range and pharmacokinetics.

Match each cultural group with its corresponding cultural practice.

11. _____ Chinese

12. _____ Hispanic

13. _____ Aboriginal

14. _____ Black and Caribbean

a. Some may seek a balance between the body and mind through the use of cold remedies or foods for "hot" illnesses, and vice versa.

b. Some may use folk medicine and have strong spiritual belief influences.

c. Some believe that opposing forces of negative (yin) and positive (yang) energies lead to illness or health, depending on which force is in balance.

d. Some believe in the balance between the body, mind, and environment to maintain health and harmony with nature.

CRITICAL THINKING AND APPLICATION

Answer the following questions on a separate sheet of paper.

15. Identify a cultural group in your area, and explore the health belief practices of that group.

    a. Are there any barriers to adequate health care?

    b. What is the attitude toward Western medicines and health treatments?

    c. What questions should you ask in your ethnocultural assessment?

CASE STUDY

Read the scenario and answer the following questions on a separate sheet of paper.

The nurse works in an outpatient treatment clinic for patients with HIV infection. During a recent staff meeting, the medical director discussed a new drug that has shown good results in clinical trials in another country. This drug has not yet been tested in Canada. She stated that she hopes to start clinical trials of that drug in the HIV clinic.

    The following week, the nurse is asked to give a new drug regimen for four patients with HIV. One of the drugs is unfamiliar to her, and when she ask about it, the medical director states, "Oh, that's the new drug I mentioned last week! One of my colleagues in that country sent me some samples, so we are going to try it here. Health Canada has already started trials in Canada. We will be comparing how these four patients do compared with four other patients who are in the same stages of HIV. The patients will not even know about this change."

1. Should the nurse give the drugs as requested? If not, what should be done to correct the situation?

2. What ethical principle(s) guide the nurse's decision?

3. One of the potential study patients, brought in by his brother, seems reluctant to answer questions and says he "does not need any drugs." Upon further questioning, the nurse finds out that he would prefer to take some home remedies that his mother has made for him. How should the nurse handle this situation?

4. When the nurse meets with potential study patients, several mention that they fear others will find out about their illness if they participate in the study. What should the nurse tell these patients?

Chapter 5

Medication Errors

CHAPTER REVIEW

Provide the best answer for each of the following.

1. A(n) _____ is defined as any preventable adverse drug event that involves inappropriate medication use by a patient or health care professional. It may or may not cause harm to the patient.

2. A(n) _____ reaction is defined as an abnormal and unexpected response to a medication, other than an allergic reaction, that is peculiar to an individual patient.

3. A(n) _____ is defined as any undesirable effect of a medication that is expected or anticipated to occur in patients who received a given medication.

4. A(n) _____ is a type of adverse drug event that is defined as any unexpected, unintended, or excessive response to a medication.

5. A(n) _____ is an undesirable occurrence related to administration of or failure to administer a prescribed medication.

6. True or false: All adverse drug reactions are adverse drug events.

7. True or false: All adverse drug events are caused by medication errors.

8. Identify six ways to avoid medication errors.

9. Name at least four classifications of medications that are considered "high alert" drugs and are often involved in errors.

10. The Institute for Safe Medication Practices (ISMP) Canada recommends that certain abbreviations be written out in full instead of using the abbreviation. For the following abbreviations in bold font, write out the full meaning of the word or phrase.

digoxin 125 **mcg** PO now	
furosemide 40 mg IV **qd**	
d/c all meds	
NPH insulin 12 **u** SQ **ac** breakfast **qd**	
garamycin otic drops 1 **gtt AD** bid	

CASE STUDY

Read the scenario and answer the following questions on a separate sheet of paper.

A nursing student discovers that she has given her patient two acetylsalicytic acid (Aspirin) tablets instead of the one-tablet daily dose that was ordered for antiplatelet effects. She is upset and talks to her fellow students, who tell her to keep quiet about it. "One extra Aspirin will not hurt your patient," they tell her.

1. What should the nursing student do first? Describe other appropriate actions after this.

2. How could the student have prevented this error?

3. Should the patient be told about it? Explain your answer.

4. If the patient was not hurt by this incident, then is it considered a medication error? Explain.

5. The student has decided to inform her instructor. The instructor helps the student complete a report to the Canadian Medication Incident Reporting and Prevention System (CMIRPS). Explain the reason for this report. Will the student's name be reported?

Chapter 6

Patient Education and Drug Therapy

CRITICAL THINKING AND APPLICATION

Answer the following questions on a separate sheet of paper.

1. The nurse is to present information regarding antihypertensive drug therapy to two patients, a 40-year-old and a 78-year-old. Describe the differences in interventions he would use in his teaching strategies related to possible alterations in thought processes and sensory-perceptual status in these two patients.

2. The nurse is to present information to a young mother on how to help her 8-year-old child use a metered-dose inhaler. Neither the mother nor her child speaks English. Discuss strategies to use in developing a teaching plan for them.

3. The nurse's patient has been taking oral antihyperglycemics for 1 month, and her blood glucose readings are still high. On assessment, the nurse discovers a possible reason for these high readings. Develop a nursing diagnosis for this patient based on the following:

   a. The patient says that no one has ever told her about required dietary restrictions.

   b. The patient tells the nurse that she only takes the medication if she feels ill.

4. For each of the following medications, develop a measurable goal and specific outcome criteria related to teaching a patient about the medication therapy. Use later chapters in the textbook for reference.

   a. Oral contraceptives

   b. Diuretic therapy with furosemide (Lasix)

   c. digoxin (Lanoxin)

   d. Transdermal nitroglycerin patches

   e. indomethacin (Apo-Indomethacin)

5. Develop a patient teaching plan for a 55-year-old patient who will be receiving warfarin sodium (Coumadin) therapy after discharge. Refer to the appropriate chapter in the text for information. Include the following:

   a. Assessment—objective and subjective data that would be needed

   b. Nursing diagnosis

   c. Planning—measurable goal and outcome criteria

d. Implementation—specific educational strategies

e. Evaluation—means for evaluating that learning had occurred

CASE STUDY

Read the scenario and answer the following questions on a separate sheet of paper.

A 77-year-old man, accompanied by his wife, visits the office for a 3-month checkup. He has been treated for hypertension and has a history of angina. While in the office, he pulls a small bottle of sublingual nitroglycerin spray from his pants pocket and states, "I never go anywhere without this." He says he "gets along okay" with his medicines at home and that it "doesn't hurt anything" if he misses a day or two of his medications. His blood pressure today is 130/92 mm Hg, pulse rate is 88 beats/min, and respiratory rate is 12 breaths/min. Previously, his blood pressure readings have been 160/98, 152/92, and 148/94 mm Hg.

After the patient is evaluated by the physician, new medication orders are written as follows:

- hydrochlorothiazide (Apo-Hydro) 25 mg tablet, once a day
- potassium chloride (Slow-K), 600 mg (1 tablet) daily
- diltiazem (Diltiazem-60) 60 mg tablet, three times a day
- lansoprazole (Apo-Lansoprazole), 15 mg capsule, before breakfast and dinner
- nitroglycerin (Mylan-Nitro sublingual spray), as needed for chest pain

1. Based on your assessment, what nursing diagnosis would you suggest for this situation?

2. State a goal and outcome criteria for your nursing diagnosis.

3. Describe the teaching strategies the nurse would use when teaching this patient about how to take his medications correctly.

4. How would the nurse evaluate the education process in this situation?

Chapter 7

Over-the-Counter Drugs and Natural Health Products

DOUBLE PUZZLE

Unscramble each of the clue words. Take the letters that appear in circles and unscramble them for the final message.

LAIREANV

RCGIAL

FEFREEVW

TS. NOJH'S TWRO

KONIGG

WAS OLTATPEM

NISGGNE

NAAHICCEE

LAOE

SOADELNEGL

CHAPTER REVIEW

Choose the best answer for each of the following.

1. Classifications of drugs commonly used as over-the-counter (OTC) remedies include which of the following? Select all that apply.
   a. Nonsteroidal anti-inflammatory drugs
   b. Cold remedies
   c. Antibiotics
   d. Smoking-deterrent systems
   e. Topical antiviral ointments
   f. Histamine-2 (H_2) blockers

2. Advantages of over-the-counter remedies include which of the following?
   a. Third-party health insurance payers usually cover the costs.
   b. Patients can feel better faster when self-medicating.
   c. There are fewer drug interactions.
   d. Patients can self-treat minor ailments and reduce physician visits.

3. In Canada, Health Canada does which of the following regarding the manufacturing of natural health products?
   a. Enforces standards of natural health product quality and safety
   b. Requires the manufacturers of natural health products to prove efficacy
   c. Sets standards for quality control
   d. Defines natural health products as dietary supplements

4. Tachyphylaxis may develop in patients who use which of the following natural health products?
   a. Aloe
   b. Echinacea
   c. Feverfew
   d. Kava

5. The nurse is admitting a patient who has a diagnosis of right lower lobe pneumonia. Upon assessment, the nurse learns that the patient is wearing an herbal aromatherapy pack on her chest. What should the nurse do first?
   a. Remove the pack immediately.
   b. Report the pack to the physician.
   c. Ask the patient about the herbal pack.
   d. Document the presence of the herbal pack.

CRITICAL THINKING AND APPLICATION

Answer the following questions on a separate sheet of paper.

6. Which natural health products mentioned in this chapter may have serious interactions with anticoagulants such as heparin and warfarin?

7. List the types of individuals who may have more frequent adverse reactions to OTC drugs.

8. List contraindications to the use of natural health products.

9. Identify an OTC product or natural health product that you (or a family member) take and review the indications, drug interactions, contraindications, and adverse effects. Did you find any concerns?

CASE STUDY

Read the scenario and answer the following questions on a separate sheet of paper.

A 30-year-old woman is in the clinic for her yearly gynecological checkup. She is not pregnant but would like to have children soon and states that she and her husband are trying to conceive. She states that she is "concerned" about her health and watches her diet and exercises regularly to stay in shape. She has a family history of heart disease but no other conditions. Her physical assessment revealed no abnormalities or health problems.

On her medical history sheet, she writes that she takes several drug and natural health products, as follows:

"Echinacea, from September to March, to prevent influenza
Adult Aspirin, one tablet every day, to prevent a heart attack
Garlic tablets twice a day for my heart
Kava tea as needed for relaxation
One glass of red wine with dinner
Valerian capsules for sleep as needed (usually three or four times a week)"

1. Are there any drug or natural health drug interactions in this listing?

2. Do any of these products have a potential for problems if used over the long term?

3. Is there any specific information on which the nurse should focus in taking the patient's history or performing an assessment, given that she is using these drugs and natural health products?

4. She tells the nurse that she thinks the natural health products are "safe" because the government would not allow them to be sold if they were not. Is this true?

5. What would the nurse emphasize when teaching her about the use of natural health products and OTC drugs?

Chapter 8

Vitamins and Minerals

CHAPTER REVIEW

Match each definition with its corresponding term.

1. _____ Specialized protein that catalyzes chemical reactions in organic matter

2. _____ A deficiency of cyanocobalamin

3. _____ A nonprotein substance that combines with a protein molecule to form an active enzyme

4. _____ A condition caused by a vitamin D deficiency that is characterized by soft, pliable bones

5. _____ An inorganic substance ingested and attached to enzymes or other organic molecules

6. _____ An organic compound essential in small quantities for normal physiological and metabolic functioning in the body

7. _____ A condition resulting from an ascorbic acid deficiency that is characterized by weakness and anemia

8. _____ An essential organic compound that can be dissolved and stored in the liver and fatty tissues

9. _____ Biologically active chemicals that make up vitamin E compounds

10. _____ A disease of the peripheral nerves caused by an inability to assimilate thiamine

11. _____ An essential organic compound that can be dissolved in water but is not stored in the body for long periods of time

12. _____ A disease resulting from a niacin or a metabolic defect that interferes with the conversion of tryptophan to niacin

a. Beriberi

b. Coenzyme

c. Enzyme

d. Fat-soluble vitamin

e. Mineral

f. Pellagra

g. Pernicious anemia

h. Rickets

i. Scurvy

j. Tocopherols

k. Vitamin

l. Water-soluble vitamin

Choose the best answer for each of the following.

13. When giving vitamins, the nurse needs to remember that certain vitamins can be toxic if consumed in excess amounts. These include which of the following? Select all that apply.
    a. vitamin A
    b. vitamin C
    c. niacin
    d. vitamin D
    e. vitamin K
    f. folic acid

14. Cindi believes that taking megadoses of vitamin C is healthy. Which of the following should the nurse tell the patient about megadoses of vitamin C?
    a. They are usually nontoxic because vitamin C is water soluble.
    b. They can produce nausea, vomiting, headache, and abdominal cramps.
    c. They can lead to scurvy-like symptoms.
    d. They may cause dangerous heart dysrhythmias.

15. If excessive amounts of water-soluble vitamins are ingested, what usually happens?
    a. The body will store them in muscle and fat tissue until needed.
    b. They are stored in the liver until needed.
    c. They circulate in the blood, bound to proteins, until needed.
    d. Excess amounts are excreted in the urine.

16. When reviewing the diet of a patient who has a calcium deficiency, the nurse recalls that efficient absorption of calcium in the diet requires adequate amounts of which of the following?
    a. magnesium
    b. Intrinsic factor
    c. Coenzymes
    d. vitamin D

CRITICAL THINKING AND APPLICATION

Answer the following questions on a separate sheet of paper.

17. Mrs. Steinman has developed vitamin D deficiency as the result of long-term use of lubricant laxatives. She is advised to take supplements for vitamin D deficiency. However, the physician also advises her to get vitamin D through more natural sources, both dietary and endogenous. "What did he mean by 'endogenous'?" she asks the nurse. Explain to Mrs. Steinman what is meant by an endogenous source, and make her a list of foods rich in vitamin D as well.

18. Ms. Nowaczinski has recently undergone an ileal resection, which is understandably affecting her digestive functions. She is experiencing some signs of malabsorption. When routine laboratory tests are performed, the nurse discovers that she is mildly anemic.

    a. What type of anemia does the nurse expect?

    b. What about her condition is contributing to this deficiency?

    c. Create a hand-held patient education card for Ms. Nowaczinski, concentrating on diet. Be sure to include a list of foods that contain the vitamin or vitamins from which she is most likely to suffer a deficiency.

19. Mr. Graham is hospitalized with severe hypocalcemia. The nurse's colleague, Jeffrey, recommends immediately beginning a rapid infusion of intravenous calcium. The physician's order requires infusion of 1% procaine. Refute or defend the rationales of both Jeffrey and Mr. Graham's physician. In either case, what should the nurse watch out for when giving intravenous calcium? Support your response with your own data.

20. Mrs. Smith will be taking iron for treatment of anemia, and her physician instructed her to take it with orange juice. She asks the nurse for an explanation of this. What does the nurse tell her?

CASE STUDY

Read the scenario and answer the following questions on a separate sheet of paper.

After Mr. Wong is treated for colitis with a broad-spectrum antibiotic, he begins to show signs of vitamin K deficiency.

1. How did this happen? How will he receive supplements?

2. What function does vitamin K serve in the human body?

3. Despite the infrequent occurrence of this deficiency, what other patient populations can sometimes be at risk for it?

4. What dietary supplements can the nurse recommend?

Chapter 9

Problematic Substance Use

Match each drug with its corresponding description.

1. _____ cocaine

2. _____ methamphetamine

3. _____ phenobarbital

4. _____ heroin

5. _____ disulfiram (Antabuse)

6. _____ nicotine

7. _____ naltrexone (ReViva)

8. _____ buproprion (Zyban)

9. _____ opium

10. _____ "roofies"

a. A nicotine-free treatment for nicotine dependence

b. Known as the "date rape" drug

c. The source plant for heroin

d. The addictive chemical in tobacco products

e. An opioid that is injected by "mainlining" or "skin popping"

f. Used in managing withdrawal from barbiturates

g. Used to deter the use of alcohol during alcohol dependence treatment

h. A stimulant that is either "snorted" through the nasal passages or injected intravenously

i. A stimulant that is popular at "raves" with college-age students

j. An opioid antagonist used for opioid misuse or dependence

Choose the best answer for each of the following.

11. A patient who has been taking disulfiram (Antabuse) therapy for 3 months has been off the therapy for 2 days. He decides to go out with friends to have a beer. What effects may he experience?
    a. No ill effects
    b. Diarrhea
    c. Vomiting
    d. Euphoria

12. Which of the following is the most common drug effect leading to abuse of opioids?
    a. Hallucinations
    b. Sleep
    c. Stimulation
    d. Relaxation and euphoria

13. Which of the following medications may be used to manage opioid withdrawal?
    a. disulfiram (Antabuse)
    b. clonidine (Catapres)
    c. methadone (Metadol)
    d. bupropion (Zyban)
    e. naltrexone (ReViva)

14. When teaching a patient about drug interactions, the nurse is aware that combining benzodiazepines with ethanol or barbiturates may lead to death due to which of the following?
    a. Cardiac dysrhythmia
    b. Convulsions
    c. Respiratory arrest
    d. Stroke

15. A patient with a known history of chronic excessive ingestion of ethanol has developed memory problems and comes to the health clinic with hard-to-believe stories of what has happened to him. The nurse recognizes that these symptoms are associated with which disorder?
    a. Cerebrovascular accident
    b. Korsakoff's psychosis
    c. Narcolepsy
    d. Bipolar disorder

CRITICAL THINKING AND APPLICATION

Answer the following questions on a separate sheet of paper.

16. Describe how nicotine is used to ease withdrawal from nicotine use. How is bupropion (Zyban) used in smoking cessation programs?

17. How is medication therapy different for mild, moderate, and severe alcohol withdrawal?

CASE STUDY

Read the scenario and answer the following questions on a separate sheet of paper.

A 19-year-old male, Mr. Chan, is admitted to the emergency department after he collapsed at a graduation party. The paramedics state that there were beer-drinking contests at the party, and it is unknown how much Mr. Chan had to drink. His friend says that Mr. Chan was upset over losing his girlfriend, and he has worried about how heavily Mr. Chan has been drinking in the past 2 weeks.

Mr. Chan is semiconscious but unable to answer questions coherently, and his speech is slurred. His blood pressure is 100/58 mm Hg, his pulse rate is 110 beats/min, and his breathing is heavy, with a respiratory rate of 16 breaths/min. He vomited on the way to the hospital.

1. Is ethanol considered a central nervous system (CNS) stimulant or depressant?

2. What are the effects of severe alcoholic intoxication on the cardiovascular and respiratory systems?

3. The patient is admitted to the medical unit for observation. For what should the nurse be observant at this time?

4. The next evening Mr. Chan is more alert but still unsteady with his gait. He says he wants to go home, but the nurse notices fine tremors of his hands. Should he be discharged at this time? Explain.

5. If Mr. Chan continues the pattern of heavy drinking, what effects could the chronic ingestion of ethanol have on his body?

Chapter 10

Photo Atlas of Drug Administration

CHAPTER REVIEW

Choose the best answer for each of the following.

1. To expel air bubbles after drawing fluid from an ampule, remove the needle, hold the syringe with the needle pointing up, and do which of the following?
   a. Draw back slightly on the plunger, tap the side of the syringe to cause bubbles to rise toward the needle, and push the plunger upward to eject air.
   b. Tap the side of the syringe to cause bubbles to rise toward the needle, draw back slightly on the plunger, and push the plunger upward to eject air.
   c. Tap the side of the syringe to cause bubbles to rise toward the needle, draw back slightly on the plunger, push the plunger upward to eject air, and eject a small amount of fluid.
   d. Draw back slightly on the plunger, tap the side of the syringe to cause bubbles to rise toward the needle, and push the plunger upward to eject air; do not eject fluid.

2. When giving intradermal injections, the nurse will remember to do which of the following?
   a. Massage the site lightly after the injection.
   b. Have the patient massage the site until the pain diminishes.
   c. Avoid massaging the site.
   d. Apply heat to the site after the injection.

3. When medication is administered by intravenous push, the correct way to occlude the intravenous line is to do which of the following?
   a. Pinch the tubing just above the injection port.
   b. Pinch the tubing at least 5 cm above the injection port.
   c. Fold the tubing just above the injection port.
   d. Do not occlude the line because it is not necessary to do so for this procedure.

4. When more than one medication is to be added to a solution, which action is correct?
   a. Use an equal volume of each medication.
   b. First assess the two drugs for compatibility.
   c. Always add the drugs at least 1 hour apart.
   d. Use the same needle for both medications.

5. When oral medications are administered, which action is correct?
   a. If a patient cannot swallow medications, crush all medications together and administer with applesauce.
   b. Give oral medications with meals to avoid gastrointestinal upset.
   c. Stay with the patient until each medication has been swallowed.
   d. Give all medications on an empty stomach to facilitate absorption.

6. When administering ear drops, which action by the nurse is correct?
   a. Press a cotton ball firmly into the ear canal after giving the drops.
   b. Have the patient sit up and tilt the head for 2 to 3 minutes.
   c. Gently massage the tragus of the ear.
   d. Have the patient remain in the side-lying position for 20 minutes.

7. Which position is correct when the nurse administers nasal drops for the frontal or maxillary sinuses?
   a. Tilt the patient's head backward and facing toward the left side.
   b. Tilt the patient's head back over the edge of the bed, with the head turned toward the side treated.
   c. Place a pillow under the patient's shoulders and tilt the head back.
   d. Tilt the patient's head to the side opposite the side treated.

8. Which of the following actions by the nurse is correct when administering drugs via a nasogastric tube?
   a. Allow the fluid to flow via gravity.
   b. Use gentle but consistent pressure when forcing the fluid into the tube.
   c. Shake the tube gently to facilitate the movement of fluid in the tube.
   d. Confirm placement of the tube after the medication is given.

9. Z-track intramuscular injections are indicated in which of the following situations?
   a. When there is insufficient muscle mass in the landmarked area
   b. Whenever massaging the area after medication administration is contraindicated
   c. With medications that are known to be irritating, painful, or staining to tissues
   d. With any injection that is given into the dorsogluteal muscle

10. When giving sublingual medications, the nurse recalls that medications given by this route have which advantage?
    a. They are immediately absorbed.
    b. They are excreted rapidly.
    c. They are metabolized immediately.
    d. They are distributed equally.

11. The dosage of a prochlorperazine (PMS-Prochlorperazine) rectal suppository is twice what has actually been ordered. The nurse's most appropriate intervention would be which of the following?
    a. Cut the suppository in half.
    b. Call the physician for clarification.
    c. Administer another type of suppository.
    d. Instruct the patient to retain the suppository for only 5 minutes.

12. Which of the following is a contraindication for the administration of rectal suppositories?
    a. Vomiting
    b. Fever
    c. Constipation
    d. Rectal bleeding

13. The nurse applies a transdermal patch. What condition must the site be in before medications are given by transdermal (skin) administration?
    a. Hairy
    b. Nonhairy
    c. Moist
    d. Within a skinfold

14. Which of the following is important to tell the patient when teaching about the instillation of nasal drops?
    a. Clear the nasal passages by blowing the nose gently before administering the medication.
    b. Clear the nasal passages by blowing the nose gently after administering the medication.
    c. Sit in the semi-Fowler position for 5 minutes after the instillation of the medication.
    d. Place the nose dropper approximately 1 cm into the nostril when instilling drops.

15. Which of the following is true regarding the administration of ophthalmic medications? Select all that apply.
    a. Have the patient look upward while instilling the medication.
    b. Instill the prescribed number of drops into the conjunctival sac.
    c. Have the patient close his or her eyes tightly after the drop has been instilled.
    d. Apply gentle pressure to the patient's nasolacrimal duct for 30 to 60 seconds after instilling the drops.
    e. Apply ointment to the conjunctival sac, starting at the outer canthus and working toward the inner canthus.

CRITICAL THINKING AND APPLICATION

Answer the following questions on a separate sheet of paper.

16. Describe how the nurse assesses the injection site for each of the following:

    a. Subcutaneous injection

    b. Intramuscular injection

    c. Intradermal injection

17. Describe the proper technique of needle insertion for each of the following:

    a. Subcutaneous injection

    b. Intramuscular injection

    c. Intradermal injection

18. The nurse is administering an intramuscular injection to his patient. After the needle enters the site, the nurse grasps the lower end of the syringe barrel with his nondominant hand and slowly pulls back on the plunger to aspirate the drug. Blood appears in the syringe. What should he do?

19. The nurse is preparing a liquid medication for a patient. How does the usual procedure change when the volume of medication required is less than 5 mL?

20. A patient has been given a new inhaler that contains 250 doses of medication. The order specifies that the patient is to take "one puff four times a day." How many days will this inhaler last before it becomes empty?

CASE STUDY

Read the scenario and answer the following questions on a separate sheet of paper.

A mother comes to a family practice office with her 2-year-old daughter and 8-month-old son. She is planning a trip abroad and needs to obtain immunizations for herself and her children before she leaves.

1. The mother and the infant each need to be given an intramuscular immunization. Describe the differences in choosing sites and giving an intramuscular injection in the mother and the infant.

2. The 2-year-old daughter has an ear infection, and the physician prescribed ear drops. What should the nurse teach the mother about giving these ear drops to her child?

3. Two days later, the mother brings the infant back to the office because she has developed a high fever. The nurse prepares to give the infant a liquid oral antipyretic and discovers that the dose is 4 mL. How does the nurse measure this medication?

4. The mother wants to add the medication to her baby's bottle. How would the nurse administer this liquid medication to the infant?

Chapter 11

Analgesic Drugs

CRITICAL THINKING CROSSWORD

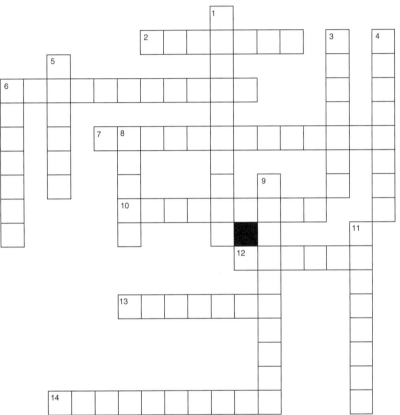

Across

2. Any drug that binds to a receptor and causes a response has _____ properties.
6. Mrs. Guo is experiencing pain and itching due to a severe case of poison ivy on the skin of her arms and legs. She is experiencing _____ pain.
7. Mr. Romano, described in 12 Across, is recovering. He requires continued pain management but is able to take less powerful doses of medication now. Every day he tells the nurse that he finds he can do "more and more normal things, even though there is still some pain there." Mr. Romano is describing his level of _____ _____. (*Two words*)

Down

1. Mr. Fernandez's drug binds to a receptor but causes the opposite effect of the type of drug discussed in 13 Across. He is taking a drug with _____ properties.
3. Mrs. Sistani has suffered back pain "for years." She says that it is worse in the late afternoon and at night but that "really, even when it lessens somewhat, it is there all the time in some form." Mrs. Sistani is experiencing _____ pain.
4. Mr. Garcia paces the floor all night, holding his side. The pain is so severe that he vomits. His wife brings him to the emergency department, where it is quickly recognized that Mr. Garcia has a kidney stone. The type of pain he has been experiencing is _____ pain.

10. Ms. Lipponen was in an automobile crash and injured her leg. In assessing the level of stimulus applied to her toe that results in a perception of pain, the nurse is testing her pain _____.

12. Mr. Romano is brought to the emergency room in tremendous pain. The emergency room team recognizes the need to immediately bring the pain under some control to make assessment, diagnosis, and treatment more manageable. After assessing that it is not contraindicated, the attending physician initiates administration of a strong and addicting pain reliever. This is no doubt a(n) _____ analgesic.

13. Ms. Tanaka is taking a drug that binds to part of a receptor and causes effects that are not as strong as those of a pure agonist. She is taking a(n) _____ agonist.

14. Mr. Birhanu is suffering the effects of withdrawal from an opioid analgesic; he has become physically dependent on the drug, and now that he no longer has access to it, he is suffering withdrawal, or opioid _____ syndrome.

5. This word is often used interchangeably with the term "opioid." _____

6. Mr. Jankowski has injured himself in a friendly basketball game with his peers after work. His wife brings him to the urgent care centre several hours later because of the pain. Mr. Jankowski is probably experiencing _____ pain.

8. Mrs. Milo had breast reduction surgery yesterday and is complaining of pain around her incisions. Mrs. Milo is experiencing _____ pain.

9. Mr. Chadwick has entered a treatment centre to help him overcome a psychological dependence on a cocaine derivative. He is seeking help for a _____ use of this drug, characterized by a continuous craving that is not pain related.

11. Mr. Vu is already taking an opioid pain reliever. When his pain increases, the drug is not as effective. He is given a second analgesic drug in addition to the first drug. "Two pain killers?" he asks the nurse. "Is that safe?" The nurse explains that the second drug is not a primary analgesic but has properties that will add to the analgesic effects of the opioid. It is being used, then, as a(n) _____ drug.

CHAPTER REVIEW

Choose the best answer for each of the following.

1. During a marathon, a runner had to drop out after 25 kilometres because of severe muscle spasms. This type of pain is classified as which of the following?
   a. Persistent pain
   b. Somatic pain
   c. Visceral pain
   d. Superficial pain

2. A 23-year-old male has been taken to the emergency department because of a suspected overdose of morphine tablets. Which drug may be used to treat this overdose?
   a. meperidine (Demerol)
   b. naproxen sodium (Anaprox)
   c. acetylsalicylic acid (Aspirin)
   d. naloxone HCl

3. An anticonvulsant drug has been ordered as part of a patient's pain management program. The purpose of the anticonvulsant in this case is to achieve which of the following?
   a. Produce sleep
   b. Prevent seizures
   c. Relieve neuropathic pain
   d. Reduce anxiety

4. Moderate to severe pain is best treated with which of the following?
   a. acetaminophen (Tylenol)
   b. Opioid antagonists
   c. Benzodiazepines
   d. Opioid analgesics

5. Which of the following should be included in an assessment before giving an opioid analgesic? Select all that apply.
   a. Blood clotting times
   b. The level of pain rated on a scale
   c. Prior analgesic use (time, type, amount, and effectiveness)
   d. Dietary history
   e. Allergies

Match each type of pain with its corresponding description.

6. _____ Acute pain

7. _____ Persistent pain

8. _____ Somatic pain

9. _____ Visceral pain

10. _____ Superficial pain

11. _____ Vascular pain

12. _____ Neuropathic pain

13. _____ Phantom pain

14. _____ Psychogenic pain

15. _____ Central pain

a. Pain that is due to psychological factors, not physical conditions or disorders

b. Pain that is thought to account for most migraine headaches

c. Pain that occurs in a body part that has been removed

d. Pain that originates from the skin or mucous membranes

e. Pain that occurs with tumours, trauma, or inflammation of the brain

f. Recurring persistent pain that is often difficult to treat

g. Pain that is sudden in onset and usually subsides when treated

h. Pain that originates from the organs or smooth muscles

i. Pain that originates from the skeletal muscles, ligaments, or joints

j. Pain that results from injury or damage to the peripheral nerve fibres

CASE STUDY

Read the scenario and answer the following questions on a separate sheet of paper.

A 58-year-old woman has been admitted for surgery to remove a small growth from her lower back, just under the skin. That evening she asks for pain medication. Upon assessment, the nurse finds that she rates her pain level as "8" and that her pain is located mainly in the immediate area around her incision. The nurse prepares to give her an intravenous dose of morphine sulfate.

1. What type of pain is she experiencing?

2. What nonpharmacological intervention may be used to reduce her pain?

3. Within 1 hour of receiving the morphine, the patient complains that her skin feels "itchy," but she cannot see any hives. What does the nurse tell her?

4. What serious adverse effect is possible if she receives too much morphine sulfate? What, if anything, can be given to treat this?

5. Two days later she is ready to be discharged to home. Her physician writes a prescription for oxycodone HCl (OxyContin) and acetominophen (Tylenol). The patient sees the label and asks why she is "only getting Tylenol" for her pain. Explain the purpose of the acetaminophen in this medication and for her pain treatment.

Chapter 12
General and Local Anaesthetics

CRITICAL THINKING CROSSWORD

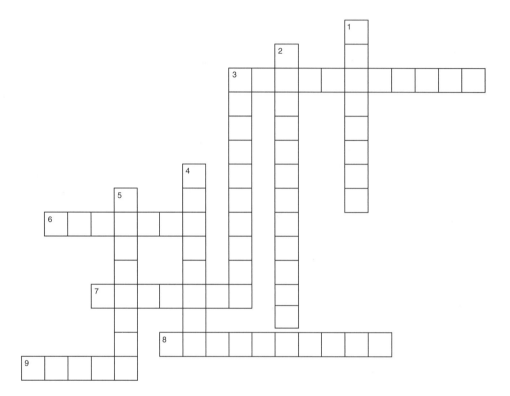

Across

3. A commonly used, long-acting, nondepolarizing neuromuscular blocking agent (NMBA).
6. Anaesthetic drugs that alter the central nervous system (CNS), resulting in loss of consciousness and deep muscle relaxation, are called _____.
7. _____ anaesthetics are applied directly to the skin and mucous membranes.
8. Drugs used in combination with anaesthetic drugs to control the adverse effects of anaesthetics.
9. Drugs that render a specific portion of the body insensitive to pain without affecting consciousness are called _____ anaesthetics.

Down

1. An anticholinergic drug given preoperatively to dry secretions.
2. A broad term for drugs that depress the CNS.
3. Anaesthetics administered directly into the CNS by various spinal injection techniques are examples of _____ anaesthetics.
4. The practice of using combinations of drugs to produce general anaesthesia, rather than using a single drug.
5. Another name for 9 Across.

CHAPTER REVIEW

Choose the best answer for each of the following.

1. Examples of adjunctive drugs used with anaesthesia include which of the following? Select all that apply.
   a. Sedative–hypnotics
   b. Anticonvulsants
   c. Anticholinergics
   d. Inhaled gas
   e. Opioid analgesics

2. Lidocaine is frequently used for which of the following?
   a. Spinal anaesthesia
   b. Local anaesthesia
   c. Intravenous anaesthesia
   d. General anaesthesia

3. The nurse monitoring a patient after surgery keeps in mind that the primary concern with use of an NMBA is which of the following?
   a. Respiratory arrest
   b. Headache
   c. Bradycardia
   d. Hypertension

4. To decrease the possibility of a headache after spinal anaesthesia, the nurse should instruct the patient to do which of the following?
   a. Sit in high Fowler's position
   b. Lie flat in bed
   c. Limit fluids
   d. Engage in activity

5. Local anaesthesia is indicated for which of the following? Select all that apply.
   a. Cardioversions
   b. Suturing a skin laceration
   c. Diagnostic procedures
   d. Long-duration surgery
   e. Dental procedures

6. A sudden elevation in body temperature in a patient who has just returned from surgery may indicate which of the following?
   a. A normal temperature change after surgery
   b. Malignant hypertension
   c. Malignant hyperthermia
   d. Fever

7. A patient is receiving an NMBA. Indicate the order in which the following areas become paralyzed once this drug is given (1 = first, 3 = last).

   a. _____ Limbs, neck, trunk muscles

   b. _____ Intercostal muscles and diaphragm

   c. _____ Small, rapidly moving muscles, such as those of the fingers and eyes

CRITICAL THINKING AND APPLICATION

Answer the following questions on a separate sheet of paper.

8. Henry is a student nurse who has assisted the anaesthesiologist in surgery on prior occasions. Today, however, he is nervous because it is a child who will undergo general anaesthesia. Why might this make Henry more nervous than usual?

9. Mr. Mbassi is being administered an NMBA while he is receiving mechanical ventilation. What is important to remember when working with him while he is receiving this therapy?

10. Mrs. Edwards will undergo cardioversion this afternoon, and the anaesthesiologist has explained to her that she will not be asleep but that she will not remember the procedure. Mrs. Edwards asks the nurse, "How can this be?" What is the nurse's explanation?

CASE STUDY

Read the scenario and answer the following questions on a separate sheet of paper.

You are a nursing student, and today you are assigned to an observation day in the operating room, with the anaesthesiologist as your contact for the day. The first case is a patient undergoing a right lower lung lobectomy to treat lung cancer. The patient has a history of paraplegia from an old automobile accident. The patient's blood pressure has been maintained at 120/72 mm Hg and the pulse has ranged from 100 to 110 beats/min during the surgery. The patient's body temperature has lowered to 35.7°C after surgery. The patient's respirations have been maintained by ventilator.

1. Before the surgery, the anaesthesiologist explained that the patient would undergo "balanced anaesthesia." What is meant by this term?

2. What is the purpose of administering the drug succinylcholine chloride (Quelicin Chloride) during anaesthesia?

3. As your patient goes to the postanaesthesia care unit (PACU), the anaesthesiologist asks you to monitor for signs of succinylcholine toxicity. Would this be of concern at this time?

4. What can be done if the patient has received too much succinylcholine?

5. Another patient is undergoing a procedure using spinal anaesthesia. Are there advantages of this type of anaesthesia over general anaesthesia?

6. In the PACU, what are the main concerns of the nurse monitoring the patient recovering from anaesthesia?

Chapter 13

Central Nervous System Depressants and Muscle Relaxants

CHAPTER REVIEW

Choose the best answer for each of the following.

1. A hypnotic is a drug that achieves which of the following?
   a. It produces sleep.
   b. It slows the destruction of dopamine.
   c. It prevents nausea and vomiting.
   d. It relaxes the patient.

2. A patient who has been taking a benzodiazepine for 5 weeks has been instructed to stop the medication. Which of the following strategies is the best way to discontinue the medication?
   a. Stop taking the drug immediately.
   b. Plan a gradual reduction in dosage.
   c. Overlap this medication with another drug.
   d. Take the medication every other day for a number of weeks.

3. A patient will be undergoing a brief surgical procedure to obtain a biopsy from a superficial mass on his arm. The nurse expects that which type of barbiturate will be used at this time?
   a. Rapid
   b. Short
   c. Intermediate
   d. Long

4. While monitoring a patient who took an overdose of barbiturates, the nurse keeps in mind that the cause of death would be which of the following?
   a. Tachycardia
   b. Hypertension
   c. Dyspnea
   d. Respiratory arrest

5. A patient with back muscle spasms is being treated with a skeletal muscle relaxant. These drugs are most effective when used with which of the following?
   a. Benzodiazepines
   b. Moist heat
   c. Physiotherapy
   d. Acetylsalicylic acid (ASA)

6. The nurse is providing care for a patient who has accidentally taken an overdose of benzodiazepines. Which drug would be used to treat this patient?
   a. a methamphetamine
   b. a xanthine
   c. flumazenil (Anexate)
   d. naloxone HCl

CRITICAL THINKING AND APPLICATION

Answer the following questions on a separate sheet of paper.

7. A 19-year-old university student is brought to the emergency department with a suspected barbiturate overdose. What symptoms would the nurse expect to see? How is overdose treated?

8. Jackie is taking benzodiazepines to treat insomnia. Today she visits the clinic and states that she is going to Europe for 2 months and wants a prescription that will allow her to take enough medication along for her entire stay. The physician declines. She is a little insulted and asks the nurse why the physician refused her request: "Does my doctor think I'm an addict or suicidal or something?" What does the nurse explain to her? What other options are possible for her?

9. Mrs. Alexander, 81 years of age, weighs significantly more than her 47-year-old daughter, yet she is given a lower dose of medication for insomnia of a similar degree. Explain. Is this a dose calculation error?

10. The nurse has been asked to take a patient history for Willem, who will be given a benzodiazepine.

    a. What conditions should the nurse ask about?

    b. What drug intake should the nurse be most concerned about?

    c. What if Willem were an infant? A great-grandfather? Would this additional information matter? Explain.

11. Mr. Shapiro is recovering from an automobile crash and has received a prescription for cyclobenzaprine HCl (Novo-Cycloprine) for painful muscle spasms.

    a. What patient teaching should Mr. Shapiro receive about this drug?

    b. What other measures should be included in addition to this drug therapy?

12. Define *tachyphylaxis* and name one drug that can cause it. Is it an advantage or a disadvantage? Explain.

CASE STUDY

Read the scenario and answer the following questions on a separate sheet of paper.

A 44-year-old woman has had problems with insomnia "off and on for a few years" and has tried over-the-counter medications, natural health products, and prescription drugs. She likes to drink a glass of wine each night before going to bed. Today she is visiting the clinic for a checkup and asks for a prescription for lorazepam (Ativan) because that was the last prescription she tried several years ago. She says she "can't understand" why the pharmacy will not refill her prescriptions for lorazepam. The physician prescribes zopiclone (Imovane) instead.

1. Why did the physician change her prescription?

2. What are the consequences of long-term use of barbiturates?

3. What interactions should she be told about while she is taking zopiclone?

4. What other patient teaching is important for this patient?

Chapter 14

Antiepileptic Drugs

CRITICAL THINKING CROSSWORD

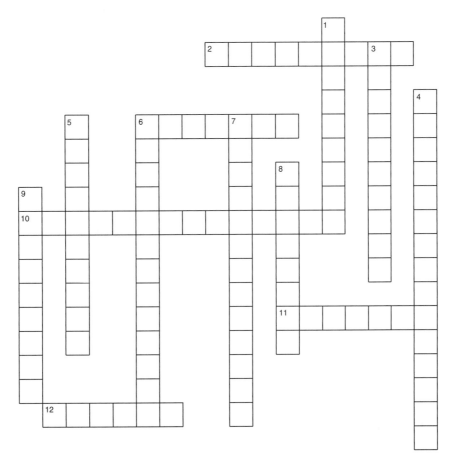

Across

2. Status epilepticus is considered a life-threatening _____.
6. A type of epilepsy with an unknown cause.
10. A potentially fatal adverse effect of valproic acid (Depakene).
11. A brief episode of abnormal electrical activity in the nerve cells of the brain.
12. Intravenously administered antiepileptic drugs should be delivered this way to avoid serious adverse effects.

Down

1. A type of epilepsy with a distinct cause.
3. An involuntary spasmodic contraction of muscles throughout the body.
4. These drugs are considered first-line drugs for the treatment of status epilepticus.
5. Another term for 6 Across.
6. A barbiturate used primarily to control tonic–clonic and partial seizures.
7. The metabolic process that occurs when the metabolism of a drug increases over time, which leads to lower-than-expected drug concentrations.
8. Recurrent episodes of convulsive seizures.
9. A first-line antiepileptic drug, the long-term use of which can cause gingival hyperplasia.

CHAPTER REVIEW

Choose the best answer for each of the following.

1. Janie has seizures characterized by temporary lapses in consciousness that last only a few seconds. Her teachers have said that she "daydreams too much." These types of seizures are known as which of the following?
   a. Simple seizures
   b. Complex seizures
   c. Partial seizures
   d. Generalized seizures

2. Which condition is a life-threatening emergency in which patients typically do not regain consciousness?
   a. Status epilepticus
   b. Tonic–clonic convulsions
   c. Epilepsy
   d. Primary epilepsy

3. Which of the following is true about the intravenous infusion of phenytoin (Dilantin)? Select all that apply.
   a. It should be injected quickly.
   b. It should be injected slowly.
   c. It should be followed by an injection of sterile saline.
   d. Continuous infusion should be avoided.

4. Which of the following is a possible adverse effect of phenobarbital therapy?
   a. Constipation
   b. Gingival hyperplasia
   c. Drowsiness
   d. Dysrhythmias

5. Which drug would be used for the treatment of status epilepticus?
   a. phenobarbital
   b. diazepam (Valium)
   c. valproic acid (Depakene)
   d. phenytoin (Dilantin)

6. A patient who is experiencing neuropathic pain tells the nurse that the physician is going to start him on a new medication that is generally used to treat seizures. The nurse anticipates that which drug will be ordered?
   a. phenobarbital
   b. phenytoin (Dilantin)
   c. gabapentin (Neurontin)
   d. lamotrigine (Lamictal)

CRITICAL THINKING AND APPLICATION

Answer the following questions on a separate sheet of paper.

7. What is meant by autoinduction in a drug? Identify at least one antiepileptic drug that undergoes autoinduction.

8. Jeremy, an 8-year-old boy, has resisted his oral doses of topiramate (Topamax), which has made adherence to the drug regimen difficult. His mother calls and says that she has found a way to get him to take it: she crushes the tablet and sprinkles it on flavoured gelatin. She is delighted. What is the nurse's response?

CASE STUDY

Read the scenario and answer the following questions on a separate sheet of paper.

Four-year-old Mattie has started preschool. Today the teacher called Mattie's mother to tell her that she noticed that Mattie seems to have a problem with "daydreaming." She explained that Mattie seemed inattentive during group work and was staring out into space several times a day. She was also worried because she saw Mattie's eyes move back and forth rapidly during these episodes. These "spells" lasted 1 to 2 minutes, and then Mattie seemed fine. The mother has brought Mattie to the pediatrician's office to have her checked. The physician suspects that Mattie is experiencing a type of seizure disorder and has ordered some diagnostic testing.

1. What type of seizure is Mattie experiencing?

2. After the diagnostic testing is performed, what medication is most likely to be prescribed for Mattie?

3. This medication comes in a syrup with a concentration of 250 mg/5 mL. What is important to teach the mother regarding administration of this medication?

4. What should the mother be taught to monitor while Mattie is taking this medication?

5. After a year, Mattie's mother is pleased that the seizures have "disappeared" and wants to take Mattie off the medication. What is the nurse's response?

Chapter 15

Antiparkinsonian Drugs

CHAPTER REVIEW

Choose the best answer for each of the following.

1. Which of the following describes a patient with Parkinson's disease who has difficulty performing voluntary movements?
   a. Akinesia
   b. Dyskinesia
   c. Chorea
   d. Dystonia

2. Which drug may be used early in the treatment of Parkinson's disease but eventually loses effectiveness and must be replaced by another drug?
   a. amantadine HCl
   b. carbidopa-levodopa (Sinemet)
   c. selegiline HCl
   d. entacapone (Comtan)

3. When teaching a patient who is taking carbidopa-levodopa (Sinemet) for Parkinson's disease, what should the nurse tell the patient about vitamin supplements?
   a. Vitamin supplements should not be taken at this time.
   b. Vitamin supplements should be taken twice a day to ensure that the patient receives enough nutrients.
   c. The patient should avoid supplements that contain vitamin B_6 (pyridoxine).
   d. The patient should not take more than the recommended amount of calcium.

4. A patient who is newly diagnosed with Parkinson's disease and beginning medication therapy with entacapone (Comtan), a catechol ortho-methyltransferase (COMT) inhibitor, asks the nurse, "How soon will improvement occur?" The nurse's best response is which of the following?
   a. "That varies from patient to patient."
   b. "You should discuss that with your physician."
   c. "You should notice a difference right away."
   d. "It may take several weeks before you notice any degree of improvement."

5. Anticholinergic drugs administered during treatment of Parkinson's disease are given to control or minimize which of the following symptoms? Select all that apply.
   a. Drooling
   b. Constipation
   c. Muscle rigidity
   d. Bradykinesia

6. A patient who has been taking carbidopa-levodopa (Sinemet) for 4 months has been instructed by the health care provider to take a "drug holiday" for 10 days. The patient should be prepared for which of the following?
   a. A reduction in symptoms of Parkinson's disease
   b. Withdrawal effects while the drug is stopped
   c. The need to take higher dosages when the drug is resumed
   d. A possible stay in the hospital during the time he is not taking the drug

CRITICAL THINKING AND APPLICATION

Answer the following questions on a separate sheet of paper.

7. Mr. Hicks is on a carbidopa/levodopa/entacapone (Stalevo) treatment regimen.

   a. What are the advantages of combining the three drugs in Mr. Hick's treatment regimen? Are there any disadvantages?

   b. What problems are avoided when carbidopa is given with levodopa?

   c. How does carbidopa work to avoid the problems in (b), above?

8. Mrs. Chatterjee, a 35-year-old new mother, has experienced slowing movements, cogwheel rigidity, and pill-rolling tremor. She has been diagnosed with Parkinson's disease, a somewhat rare occurrence in someone her age. In addition to the usual history questions, what must the nurse ask in anticipation of dopaminergic therapy in Mrs. Chatterjee's specific situation?

9. Jane, age 45, is taking benztropine mesylate (PMS-Benztropine) in addition to a dopaminergic drug for Parkinson's disease. Her 76-year-old neighbour comments that he cannot take benztropine because it is too risky for his heart and kidneys. Jane calls and asks why this is not a concern in her case. What does the nurse say?

CASE STUDY

Read the scenario and answer the following questions on a separate sheet of paper.

Alexander, a 54-year-old man, has been diagnosed with Parkinson's disease and is about to start drug therapy. His symptoms are mild, yet he has some akinesia that interferes with his ability to type at work. The physician explains that Alexander may have to take a variety of drugs as the disease progresses.

1. What is the underlying pathological defect of Parkinson's disease?

2. What is the aim of drug therapy for Parkinson's disease?

3. The first drugs prescribed for Alexander are amantadine HCl along with levodopa–carbidopa (Sinemet CR). What is the purpose of taking amantadine at this time?

4. The physician tells Alexander that the amantadine may be helpful in the early stages but will need to be changed at a later date. Why is this true?

5. What is the "on-off phenomenon" that may occur with the use of levodopa? How does carbidopa affect this phenomenon?

Chapter 16

Psychotherapeutic Drugs

CHAPTER REVIEW

Choose the best answer for each of the following.

1. Patients taking the newer antipsychotic drugs such as quetiapine fumarate (Seroquel) should be cautioned about which problem when beginning this therapy?
   a. Mood swings
   b. Diarrhea
   c. Postural hypotension
   d. Anorexia

2. When giving hydroxyzine HCl intramuscularly, what measures should be taken?
   a. Use the Z-track method.
   b. Use a large-gauge needle.
   c. Apply an ice pack to the site for 20 minutes.
   d. Divide the dose into two injections.

3. Leslie's husband Frank has been started on antidepressant therapy. She asks the nurse, "How long will it take for him to feel better?" What should the nurse respond?
   a. "Well, depression rarely responds to medication therapy."
   b. "He should be feeling better in a few days."
   c. "It may take 4 to 6 weeks before you see an improvement."
   d. "You may not see any effects for several months."

4. Extrapyramidal effects of drugs include which of the following? Select all that apply.
   a. Tremors
   b. Elation and a sense of well-being
   c. Painful muscle spasms
   d. Motor restlessness
   e. Bradycardia

5. The nurse instructs a patient who is undergoing therapy with monoamine oxidase inhibitors (MAOIs) to avoid tyramine-containing foods. What medical emergency may occur if the patient eats these foods while taking MAOIs?
   a. Gastric hemorrhage
   b. Toxic shock
   c. Cardiac arrest
   d. Severe hypertensive crisis

Match each term with its corresponding definition or description.

6. _____ sertraline HCl (Zoloft)

7. _____ Tyramine

8. _____ Tricyclics

9. _____ Psychosis

10. _____ Mania

11. _____ diazepam (Vivol)

12. _____ amitriptyline HCl

13. _____ risperidone (Risperdal)

14. _____ Benzodiazepines

15. _____ lithium carbonate (Duralith)

16. _____ Anxiety

17. _____ Affective disorders

18. _____ Depression

19. _____ phenelzine sulfate (Nardil)

20. _____ Bipolar affective disorder

a. The unpleasant state of mind in which unreal or imagined dangers are anticipated or exaggerated

b. A state characterized by an expansive emotional state (including symptoms of extreme excitement and elation) and hyperactivity

c. A group of psychotropic drugs prescribed to alleviate anxiety

d. Emotional disorders characterized by changes in mood

e. A major psychological disorder characterized by episodes of mania or hypomania, cycling with depression

f. Classified as a monoamine oxidase inhibitor (MAOI)

g. Patients taking MAOIs need to be taught to avoid foods that contain this substance

h. Antidepressant drugs that block reuptake of amine neurotransmitters

i. An abnormal emotional state characterized by exaggerated feelings of sadness, melancholy, and worthlessness out of proportion to reality

j. A frequently prescribed benzodiazepine

k. The most widely used tricyclic antidepressant

l. An atypical antipsychotic drug used to treat schizophrenia

m. A second-generation antidepressant

n. A main treatment for mania

o. A term used to describe a major emotional disorder that impairs the mental function of the affected individual to the extent that the individual cannot participate in day-to-day activities

CRITICAL THINKING AND APPLICATION

Answer the following questions on a separate sheet of paper.

21. Viktor, a 26-year-old unemployed electrician, is brought to the emergency department by his sister. He is extremely drowsy and confused, his breathing is slow and shallow, and he smells strongly of whiskey. His sister tells the nurse that Viktor has been seeing a psychiatrist for his "anxiety."

    a. What does the nurse suspect might be wrong with Viktor?

    b. How will he likely be treated?

22. Mr. Delvecchio, a 49-year-old restaurant owner, has been prescribed the MAOI phenelzine sulfate (Nardil). After the physician leaves the room but before the nurse has a chance to discuss Mr. Delvecchio's medication regimen with him, he turns to his wife and says, "I'm sure this medicine will work. Let's have a bottle of wine tonight to celebrate."

    a. What should the nurse say?

    b. A few weeks later, Mr. Delvecchio is brought to the emergency department with a severe headache, stiff neck, sweating, and elevated blood pressure. His wife says his symptoms started a few minutes after they ate at their restaurant. What is wrong with Mr. Delvecchio and what probably caused it?

23. Beth has been diagnosed with depression. Why might the physician prescribe a second-generation antidepressant instead of a first-generation antidepressant?

24. A young adult has been admitted to the emergency department with a suspected overdose of an antidepressant. The physicians are monitoring his cardiac status closely. Why is this?

CASE STUDY

Read the scenario and answer the following questions on a separate sheet of paper.

Gene, a 38-year-old businessman, mentions during a checkup that he has felt anxious and upset over the past few months. He discusses the pressures of his business and states that he has had trouble sleeping at night, which makes him more irritable. Lately he has been worried over a contract proposal that will take place in a few months. The physician gives him a prescription for alprazolam (Xanax), 0.25 mg three times a day.

1. Gene is concerned about potential adverse effects of this medication. What should the nurse tell him?

2. What other measures should be taken for Gene at this time?

3. After 3 months, Gene is back in the office for a follow-up appointment. He is upset because a friend told him about another friend who was on that same medication but died due to an overdose. Gene wants to stop taking the alprazolam immediately. Is this recommended? If not, why not?

4. What are the symptoms of alprazolam overdose, and what is the antidote, if any?

5. Six months later, Gene is no longer taking alprazolam but comes back to the office because he still feels anxious. The physician gives him a prescription for buspirone HCl (Buspar), 30 mg twice a day. Gene questions why he is given a different drug. What are the advantages, if any, of taking buspirone instead of alprazolam?

Chapter 17

Central Nervous System Stimulant Drugs

CHAPTER REVIEW

Choose the best answer for each of the following.

1. Which of the following is true about sibutramine hydrochloride monohydrate (Meridia)?
   a. It is a serotonin receptor agonist.
   b. It is indicated for appetite stimulation in patients with anorexia nervosa.
   c. It is available as an over-the-counter drug.
   d. It should not be used with other drugs that elevate serotonin.

2. Which of the following are results of stimulation of the central nervous system (CNS) by stimulant drugs? Select all that apply.
   a. Increased fatigue
   b. Decreased drowsiness
   c. Increased respiration
   d. Bradycardia
   e. Euphoria

3. Caffeine should be avoided by patients who have a history of which of the following?
   a. Cardiac dysrhythmias
   b. Asthma
   c. Diabetes mellitus
   d. Gallbladder disease

4. Serotonin agonists are newer CNS stimulants used to treat which of the following?
   a. Attention deficit hyperactivity disorder (ADHD)
   b. Hypertension
   c. Migraine headaches
   d. Narcolepsy

5. The physician has ordered orlistat (Xenical). The nurse recognizes that this drug is used to treat which of the following?
   a. Anorexia
   b. Malnutrition
   c. Narcolepsy
   d. Obesity

6. When a child is taking drugs for ADHD, the nurse should instruct the caregivers to closely monitor the child for which of the following?
   a. Blood glucose levels
   b. Physical growth, especially weight
   c. Grades at school
   d. Respiratory rates

CRITICAL THINKING AND APPLICATION

Answer the following questions on a separate sheet of paper.

7. Stacey, age 35, reports that she experiences a continuous daytime tendency to fall asleep, with multiple irresistible nap episodes. She falls asleep unexpectedly at work and in class.

   a. What is wrong with Stacey?

   b. What might be the drug of choice for Stacey?

   c. Describe the therapeutic effects of such drugs.

   d. Develop a patient teaching plan for Stacey. Offer guidelines for (i) dosage alterations and (ii) substances she might be wise to avoid.

8. Five-year-old Jeffrey is taking atomoxetine (Strattera) HCl for ADHD. What specific precautions must be taken with children who are taking drugs for ADHD? Why?

9. What nutritional counselling is needed for the patient taking orlistat (Xenical)?

10. Sadie experiences migraine headaches approximately four times a year and has a new prescription for a triptan antimigraine medication. She tells the nurse that she hopes that the medication will prevent her "awful headaches." What does the nurse tell her?

CASE STUDY

Read the scenario and answer the following questions on a separate sheet of paper.

Nancy, a 44-year-old accountant, has had an increasing number of headaches in the past year. When she has these headaches, she often is nauseated and vomits. She has been to her physician, who has ordered several diagnostic tests. As a result, Nancy has been diagnosed with migraine headaches and will be given a prescription for a serotonin agonist.

1. How do serotonin agonists work in the treatment of migraine headaches?

2. What dosage form(s) would be helpful for Nancy's situation?

3. If the physician decides to write a prescription for sumatriptan succinate (Imitrex DF), Nancy's history should be assessed for which conditions?

4. What foods may be associated with the development of migraine headaches?

5. What else should be included in the therapy for Nancy's migraine headaches?

Chapter 18

Adrenergic Drugs

CHAPTER REVIEW

Choose the best answer for each of the following.

1. Which of the following is another name for adrenergic drugs?
   a. Anticholinergic drugs
   b. Parasympathetic drugs
   c. Central nervous system drugs
   d. Sympathomimetic drugs

2. Adrenergic drugs produce which of the following effects? Select all that apply.
   a. Urinary retention
   b. Glycogenolysis
   c. Decreased respiratory rate
   d. Increased heart rate

3. The nurse is aware that adrenergic drugs may be used to treat which of the following conditions? Select all that apply.
   a. Asthma
   b. Glaucoma
   c. Hypertension
   d. Nasal congestion
   e. Seizures
   f. Nausea and vomiting

4. Tina is allergic to bees and has just been stung. She reaches for her bee-sting kit, which would most likely contain which of the following?
   a. epinephrine
   b. methylphenidate HCl (Biphentin)
   c. dopamine
   d. norepinephrine

5. Sandra, age 13, was diagnosed with asthma 2 years ago. Today her physician wants to start salmeterol (Serevent Diskus) administered via inhaler. The nurse needs to remember to include which of the following when teaching Sandra and her family about this drug?
   a. "It should be taken at the first sign of an asthma attack."
   b. "The dosage is two puffs every 4 hours or any time needed for asthma attacks."
   c. "Don't use this for an asthma attck; it is supposed to help with long-term management of your symptoms."
   d. "Be sure to use your steroid inhaler first."

CRITICAL THINKING AND APPLICATION

Answer the following questions on a separate sheet of paper.

6. Three-year-old Kyle is taking Children's Advil Cold Suspension that contains ibuprofen and pseudoephedrine HCl. How does this drug work to promote easier nasal breathing for Kyle?

7. Mr. LaFave, who has had a history of problems with a hormonal imbalance, has been admitted for septic shock, and the physician prescribes dopamine. However, something tells the nurse that Mr. LaFave's eligibility for this drug should be double-checked. What makes the nurse think to do this?

8. Mr. Ganaden and Mr. Coetzee are both on dopamine infusions. Mr. Ganaden's infusion is a low infusion rate, and Mr. Coetzee's is a high infusion rate. Why might these infusion rates be different?

9. A patient in the critical care unit (CCU) received a dose of epinephrine that is too high. For what should the nurse monitor and what should the nurse expect to do for this patient?

10. Derk, a 49-year-old construction worker, is in the urgent care centre for treatment of a leg laceration. Just after receiving an intravenous antibiotic, he starts to wheeze and says, "Oh, I just remembered. I'm allergic to penicillin!"

   a. What is happening?

   b. What should the nurse do first?

   c. What drug do you think will be given in this situation?

CASE STUDY

Read the scenario and answer the following questions on a separate sheet of paper.

Sixteen-year-old Maureen, who plays soccer on her high-school team, has been treated for asthma for a year. Her symptoms have been controlled with an inhaled steroid and occasional use of a salbutamol sulfate (Ventolin HFA) metered-dose inhaler. This afternoon, though, her mother brings her into the urgent care centre because Maureen has had trouble "getting her breath" after a particularly rough game. Maureen complains of a feeling of "tightness" in her chest and wants to sit up. She appears anxious and has a nonproductive cough. Her respiratory rate is 28 breaths/min, and her peak expiratory flow is 70% of normal. Chest auscultation reveals a short inspiratory period with prolonged expiratory wheezes in both lungs.

1. The physician orders salbutamol via nebulizer. What should the nurse assess before, during, and after giving this medication?

2. Why is salbutamol given via inhalation rather than orally?

3. After the nebulizer medication treatment is completed, Maureen complains of feeling "shaky and jittery." What does the nurse tell her?

4. The physician gives Maureen a prescription for a salmeterol (Serevent Diskus) inhaler. What is important to teach Maureen and her mother about this medication?

Chapter 19

Adrenergic-Blocking Drugs

CHAPTER REVIEW

Choose the best answer for each of the following.

1. Adrenergic blockade at the α-adrenergic receptors leads to which of the following effects? Select all that apply.
   a. Vasodilation
   b. Decreased blood pressure
   c. Increased blood pressure
   d. Constriction of the pupil
   e. Tachycardia

2. The nurse discovers that the intravenous infusion of a patient who has been receiving an intravenous vasopressor has infiltrated. The nurse will expect which drug to be used to reverse the effects of the vasopressor in the infiltrated area?
   a. phentolamine mesylate (Rogitine)
   b. prazosin HCl (Minipress)
   c. ergotamine tartrate
   d. metoprolol tartrate (Betaloc)

3. Delia, who has migraine headaches, is being evaluated. One potential treatment is ergotamine tartrate and caffeine (Cafergot) tablets. Which of the following would be a contraindication to the use of Cafergot?
   a. Asthma
   b. Hypertension
   ç. Pregnancy
   d. Hypothyroidism

4. Mr. Annan has been given terazosin hydrochloride (Hytrin) as treatment for benign prostatic hypertrophy. What instruction is important to include when teaching him about the effects of this medication?
   a. Avoid caffeine.
   b. Change position slowly to avoid orthostatic changes.
   c. Watch for weight loss of 1 kg within 2 weeks.
   d. Take extra supplements of calcium.

5. Cheri, who has been taking a β-blocker for almost 6 months, tells the nurse that she wants to stop taking this medication. The nurse's best response is which of the following?
   a. "No, there are no ill effects if this medication is stopped."
   b. "There should be only minimal effects if you stop taking this medication."
   c. "You may experience orthostatic hypotension if you stop this medication abruptly."
   d. "If you stop this medication suddenly, there is a possibility you may experience chest pain or rebound hypertension."

CRITICAL THINKING AND APPLICATION

Answer the following questions on a separate sheet of paper.

6. Mrs. Summer, a patient on the nurse's hospital floor, is receiving a dopamine intravenous infusion. When the nurse first comes on the night shift, she seems fine. However, the next time he checks on her, he notices that the intravenous line has dislodged and the infusion has infiltrated. What could happen as a result? Is this serious? What kind of treatment do you recommend? Describe the unusual injection process and its rationale.

7. Mr. Cortis has had a myocardial infarction (MI). He is told that he will be prescribed a "cardioprotective drug." He asks the nurse to explain. Why can some β-blockers be said to "protect" the heart?

8. Ms. Clarkson has been prescribed a β-blocker. She is about to be released from hospital, but first her nurse gives her instructions about taking her apical pulse for 1 full minute, as well as her blood pressure. Why? What should she be looking for? Is there anything she should be instructed to report to her physician?

9. Mr. Sniders, a 78-year-old widower, has a new prescription for prazosin HCl (Minipress) because of a new diagnosis of benign prostatic hypertrophy. What concern, if any, is there with this drug? What teaching will he need?

CASE STUDY

Read the scenario and answer the following questions on a separate sheet of paper.

Bruce, a 58-year-old accountant, is in hospital after having an MI. The physician has told him that damage to his heart was minimal, and the patient has started post-MI rehabilitation and education. The patient has discussed having to "mend his ways" because in addition to the MI, he has had asthma for years that has been managed poorly. The physician discusses starting Bruce on a β-blocker to "protect his heart" and gives him a prescription for atenolol (Tenormin).

1. What type of β-blocker is appropriate for Bruce, and why?

2. Discuss how atenolol helps in this situation.

3. What adverse effects should he be taught about when starting this medication?

4. At his 3-month checkup, Bruce tells the nurse that he wants to stop taking the medication. Should this medication be stopped abruptly?

Chapter 20

Cholinergic Drugs

CHAPTER REVIEW

Match each definition with its corresponding term. (Note: Not all terms will be used.)

1. _____ Antidote for overdose of a cholinergic drug

2. _____ Cholinergic drugs that act by making more acetylcholine (ACh) available at the receptor site, which allows ACh to bind to and stimulate the receptor

3. _____ Cholinergic drugs that bind to cholinergic receptors and activate them

4. _____ Receptors located postsynaptically in the effector organs (smooth muscle, cardiac muscle, the glands) supplied by the parasympathetic fibres

5. _____ Receptors located in the ganglia of the parasympathetic nervous system (PSNS) and the sympathetic nervous system (SNS)

6. _____ A description of the action of the PSNS

7. _____ The neurotransmitter responsible for the transmission of nerve impulses to the effector cells in the PSNS

8. _____ The enzyme responsible for breaking down ACh

a. cholinesterase

b. muscarinic

c. catecholamine

d. "fight-or-flight"

e. "rest and digest"

f. direct-acting cholinergic drugs

g. indirect-acting cholinergic drugs

h. atropine

i. acetylcholine

j. nicotinic

Choose the best answer for each of the following.

9. The desired effects of cholinergic drugs come from stimulation of which receptors?
   a. Cholinergic
   b. Nicotinic
   c. Muscarinic
   d. Ganglionic

10. The undesired effects of cholinergic drugs come from stimulation of which receptors?
    a. Cholinergic
    b. Nicotinic
    c. Muscarinic
    d. Ganglionic

11. When a patient mentions bethanechol chloride (Duvoid) when asked about his medication history, the nurse recognizes that this drug is used for the treatment of which of the following?
    a. Diarrhea
    b. Urinary retention
    c. Urinary incontinence
    d. Bladder spasms

12. When caring for a patient with a diagnosis of myasthenia gravis, the nurse can expect that which of the following drugs is being used for symptomatic treatment of this disease?
    a. bethanechol chloride (Duvoid)
    b. entacapone (Comtan)
    c. donepezil HCl (Aricept)
    d. pyridostigmine bromide (Mestinon)

13. Annie, who is 62 years old, has started taking donepezil HCl (Aricept) for early stages of Alzheimer's disease. Her daughter expresses relief that "there is finally a pill to cure Alzheimer's disease." The nurse's best response would be which of the following?
    a. "She should expect reversal of symptoms within a few days."
    b. "The dosage should be increased if no improvement is noted."
    c. "This drug may help to improve symptoms, but it is not intended as a cure."
    d. "Yes, it has been a great help for many patients."

14. A patient has received an inadvertant overdose of a cholinergic drug. Early signs of a cholinergic crisis would include which of the following? Select all that apply.
    a. Dry mouth
    b. Salivation
    c. Flushing of the skin
    d. Abdominal cramps
    e. Constipation
    f. Dyspnea

15. The nurse will prepare to give which drug to a patient who is experiencing a cholinergic crisis?
    a. atropine sulfate
    b. memantine HCl (Ebixa)
    c. donepezil (Aricept)
    d. physostigmine

CRITICAL THINKING AND APPLICATION

Answer the following questions on a separate sheet of paper.

16. List the effects of cholinergic poisoning by using the acronym SLUDGE.

17. Mrs. Sibanda has recently had abdominal surgery and is resting well, except that she is unable to void. She has some distention in her lower abdomen over the symphysis pubis.

    a. What drug is likely to be the drug of choice?

    b. Mrs. Sibanda is still unable to void. Her urinary retention worsens and becomes painful, and when her physician is contacted, he recommends radiography to determine whether a stone is present in her urinary tract; his suspicions are confirmed. How much can the physician increase her dosage of the above drug?

18. Mr. Keegan has been determined to have a high potential for a negative reaction to the cholinergic prescribed to him. However, his physician believes that the potential benefits are worth the risk.

    a. For what reaction should the nurse be closely monitoring Mr. Keegan?

    b. In addition to close monitoring, what else can the nurse do to be prepared?

19. Ms. Bethke has recently been diagnosed with myasthenia gravis and is taking medication for the treatment of symptoms associated with the disease. She asks the nurse, "How much success can I expect?"

    a. What will the nurse say?

    b. What kind of negative effects should she report to a physician?

CASE STUDY

Read the scenario and answer the following questions on a separate sheet of paper.

Arthur, a 68-year-old retired banker, has been diagnosed with early-stage Alzheimer's disease. He has remained active in his church activities and likes to golf every week. He is in the office today with his son and is asking about the "new drugs that are available to reverse Alzheimer's disease." Arthur has had no serious health problems except for a mild case of hepatitis A 1 year ago.

1. What drugs are available to "reverse Alzheimer's disease"? Explain.

2. The physician is considering either galantamine hydrobromide (Reminyl) or rivastigmine (Exelon) for Arthur. Is there anything in his history that may influence the choice of medication used for Arthur?

3. Describe the different mechanisms of action of direct-acting and indirect-acting cholinergic-blocking drugs.

4. Arthur is given a prescription for rivastigmine. What adverse effects should be expected, and what should he and his son be told regarding ways to manage these adverse effects?

5. Another drug used for the management of Alzheimer's disease is memantine (Ebixa). Describe the action and potential effect of this drug. Is it an option for Arthur?

Chapter 21

Cholinergic-Blocking Drugs

CHAPTER REVIEW

Choose the best answer for each of the following.

1. Before giving an anticholinergic drug, the nurse should check the patient's history for which of the following?
   a. Glaucoma
   b. Osteoporosis
   c. Thyroid disease
   d. Diabetes mellitus

2. Adverse effects to expect from anticholinergic drugs include which of the following? Select all that apply.
   a. Dilated pupils
   b. Constricted pupils
   c. Dry mouth
   d. Urinary retention
   e. Urinary frequency
   f. Diarrhea

3. In reviewing the medication orders for a newly admitted patient, the nurse recognizes that an indication for atropine sulfate includes which of the following?
   a. Myasthenia gravis
   b. Reduction of secretions preoperatively
   c. Tachycardia due to sinoatrial node defects
   d. Narrow-angle glaucoma

4. During patient teaching for a 70-year-old man who will be taking an anticholinergic drug, the nurse should reinforce that this medication places the patient at higher risk for which of the following?
   a. Angina
   b. Fluid overload
   c. Heat stroke
   d. Hypothermia

5. Mellie, a 28-year-old woman, is preparing to take a cruise and has asked for a prescription for motion sickness. The physician orders transdermal scopolamine (Transderm-V) patches. The nurse should include which statement when teaching the patient about this drug?
   a. "The patch can be applied anywhere on the upper body."
   b. "Apply the patch 4 to 5 hours before travel."
   c. "Apply the patch just before boarding the ship."
   d. "Be sure to change the patch daily."

CRITICAL THINKING AND APPLICATION

Answer the following questions on a separate sheet of paper.

6. A patient is given atropine sulfate before surgery. Describe how this drug is helpful during the perioperative period. What other drug can be used for this purpose?

7. Mr. Aziz is brought into the emergency department conscious but with an overdose of a cholinergic blocker.

   a. Describe how Mr. Aziz will be treated.

   b. How should the nurse respond if Mr. Aziz begins having hallucinations related to the overdose?

8. Mr. Hansen is taking dicyclomine HCl (Bentylol) for irritable bowel syndrome. He calls the clinic and tells the nurse that he would like to get his doctor's permission to take an antihistamine for his cold. What drug interactions might he expect?

9. How does atropine work in the following situations?

   a. A patient is experiencing severe bradycardia, with a heart rate of 38 beats/min, and he is losing consciousness.

   b. A pilot has been exposed to an organophosphate insecticide in an industrial accident.

CASE STUDY

Read the scenario and answer the following questions on a separate sheet of paper.

Mrs. Walsh, age 62, is in the outpatient clinic today for a physical. During history taking, she admits to having a "terrible problem" with her bladder. She describes having sudden urges to urinate and is "ashamed to say" that, at times, she has lost control of her bladder. She has had no other health issues except for "some eye problems" off and on for the past year. The physician is considering starting Mrs. Walsh on tolterodine L-tartrate (Detrol).

1. What are the contraindications for this medication? Are there any potential concerns given Mrs. Walsh's history?

2. What are the advantages of using tolterodine over other drugs with similar actions?

3. Mrs. Walsh enjoys working outside in her yard. What special precautions should she take?

4. After a week of therapy, she calls the clinic to complain of a dry mouth. She says she did not think this was supposed to happen with this drug. What advice does the nurse give to her?

Chapter 22

Positive Inotropic Drugs

CHAPTER REVIEW

Choose the best answer for each of the following.

1. When monitoring patients who are taking digoxin, the nurse keeps in mind that the serum digoxin level should be which of the following?
   a. 0.1 to 0.5 ng/mL
   b. 0.5 to 2.0 ng/mL
   c. 2.0 to 5.0 ng/mL
   d. 5.0 to 8.4 ng/mL

2. A patient is experiencing digitalis toxicity. The nurse would expect an order for which drug?
   a. vitamin K
   b. atropine
   c. digoxin immune Fab
   d. potassium

3. Before giving oral digoxin, the nurse discovers that the patient's radial pulse is 55 beats/min. The nurse's next action should be to do which of the following?
   a. Give the dose.
   b. Delay the dose until later.
   c. Hold the dose and notify the physician.
   d. Check the apical pulse for 1 minute.

4. Which statement regarding digoxin therapy and potassium levels is correct?
   a. Low potassium levels increase the chance of digoxin toxicity.
   b. High potassium levels increase the chance of digoxin toxicity.
   c. Digoxin reduces the excretion of potassium in the kidneys.
   d. Digoxin promotes the excretion of potassium in the kidneys.

5. When infusing milrinone, the nurse should keep in mind which of the following?
   a. The medication should be mixed in saline before administration.
   b. The true colour of intravenous amrinone is clear yellow.
   c. The drug may cause reddish discolouration of the extremities.
   d. Hypertension is the primary effect seen with excessive doses.

6. When caring for a patient who is taking digoxin, the nurse should monitor for signs and symptoms of toxicity, including which of the following? Select all that apply.
   a. Anorexia
   b. Diarrhea
   c. Visual changes
   d. Nausea and vomiting
   e. Headache
   f. Bradycardia

CRITICAL THINKING AND APPLICATION

Answer the following questions on a separate sheet of paper.

7. The nurse is caring for Mrs. Chin, who is undergoing cardiac glycoside therapy. She begins to vomit and complains of a headache and fatigue. Diagnostic studies reveal short episodes of ventricular tachycardia on the ECG and a serum potassium level of 6 mmol/L. What action might the nurse expect to be taken?

8. Mr. Ali has atrial fibrillation and flutter, and the physician initially prescribes digoxin intravenously at 1.5 mg/day. What is the purpose of this dosage, and how does it compare with the dosage on which Mr. Ali will be maintained?

9. How does the concept of a therapeutic window relate to the monitoring of patients taking cardiac glycosides?

10. While monitoring Mr. Ferris after oral digoxin administration, the nurse notes increased urinary output, decreased dyspnea and fatigue, and constipation. Mr. Ferris complains to the nurse that if he were allowed to eat bran as often as he used to, he would not be constipated. What do the nurse's findings indicate? What is her response to Mr. Ferris?

11. Mr. Montgomery is experiencing heart failure that has not responded well to diuretic-and-digoxin therapy. The physician changes his medication to milrinone lactate.

    a. What effect does milrinone lactate have on cardiac muscle contractility and the blood vessels?

    b. What advantage does this phosphodiesterase inhibitor have over the cardiac glycosides?

    c. What is the most worrisome adverse effect of milrinone lactate?

CASE STUDY

Read the scenario and answer the following questions on a separate sheet of paper.

A 68-year-old woman is admitted to the hospital with a diagnosis of mild left-sided heart failure. At rest she is comfortable, but she has noticed that she has symptoms when she tries to get dressed or do simple housework. She becomes short of breath with activity, tires easily but cannot sleep at night, and feels "generally irritable." She also has diffuse bilateral crackles that do not clear with coughing and a third heart sound. She has slight pedal edema. The physician has ordered therapy with intravenous digoxin (Lanoxin).

1. Digoxin has several effects. Explain the meaning of each of the following:

    a. Positive inotropic effect

    b. Negative chronotropic effect

    c. Negative dromotropic effect

2. As a result of these effects, what would the nurse expect to see with regard to each of the following?

    a. Stroke volume

    b. Venous blood pressure and vein engorgement

    c. Coronary circulation

    d. Diuresis

3. After 3 days of therapy she complains of feeling nauseated and has no appetite. She also wonders why the lights are so bright and blurry. Her radial pulse rate is 52 beats/min. When the nurse checks the result of her laboratory work, he notes that her digoxin level from that morning is 3.5 ng/mL. What should the nurse do?

Chapter 23

Antidysrhythmic Drugs

CHAPTER REVIEW

Choose the best answer for each of the following.

1. The antidysrhythmic drug lidocaine HCl is used mainly to treat which of the following?
   a. Atrial fibrillation
   b. Bradycardia
   c. Complete heart block
   d. Ventricular dysrhythmias

2. When monitoring the patient who is taking quinidine sulfate, the nurse recognizes that which of the following is a possible adverse effect of this drug?
   a. Weakness
   b. Tachycardia
   c. Gastrointestinal upset
   d. Hypertension

3. When administering amiodarone HCl (Cordarone), the nurse should monitor for which of the following adverse effects?
   a. Pulmonary toxicity
   b. Hypertension
   c. Urinary retention
   d. Visual halos

4. A primary use of verapamil HCl (Covera) is to treat which of the following conditions?
   a. Cardiac asystole
   b. Heart block
   c. Ventricular dysrhythmia, including premature ventricular contractions
   d. Recurrent paroxysmal supraventricular tachycardia (PSVT)

5. A patient is experiencing a rapid dysrhythmia, and the nurse is preparing to administer adenosine (Adenocard). Which is the correct administration technique for this drug?
   a. It should be given as a fast intravenous push.
   b. It should be given intravenously, slowly over 5 minutes.
   c. It should be taken with food or milk.
   d. It should be given as an intravenous drip infusion.

6. If a drug has a prodysrhythmic effect, then the nurse must monitor the patient for which of the following?
   a. Decreased heart rate
   b. New dysrhythmias
   c. A decrease in dysrhythmias
   d. Reduced blood pressure

7. **Match the site to its correct intrinsic rate.**

   a. Sinoatrial node: _____   (1) 40–60 beats/min

   b. Atrioventricular node: _____   (2) 40 or fewer beats/min

   c. Purkinje fibres: _____   (3) 60–100 beats/min

CRITICAL THINKING AND APPLICATION

Answer the following questions on a separate sheet of paper.

8. Mr. Killian, who has been diagnosed with hypertension, is hospitalized after a myocardial infarction (MI).

   a. To reduce the risk of sudden cardiac death in Mr. Killian, the physician prescribes a drug from which class? Why?

   b. How would a history of asthma in Mr. Killian affect the drug choice?

9. Mr. al-Hillal has a life-threatening ventricular tachycardia that has been resistant to treatment, and the physician has now prescribed what she calls a "last resort" drug. To what drug is she referring, and why is it considered a drug of last resort?

10. Mr. Kowalski is a 50-year-old teacher being treated with lidocaine after an MI.

    a. Mr. Kowalski is upset and says that he hates injections; he wants to know why he can't just take a pill. What does the nurse tell him?

    b. If Mr. Kowalski has a history of cirrhosis, would the dosage of the lidocaine be affected?

11. Mrs. Inez calls the health clinic complaining of chest pain and dizziness. She says she cannot remember whether she took her quinidine sulfate (Apo-Quin-G) yesterday and wants to know whether she should take two doses today, especially because she is feeling so bad. What does the nurse tell Mrs. Inez?

CASE STUDY

Read the scenario and answer the following questions on a separate sheet of paper.

Jack, age 39, is taking diltiazem HCl (Apo-Diltiaz) as part of treatment for occasional PSVT. He also has a history of seizures.

1. How do calcium channel blockers such as diltiazem work?

2. What therapeutic effects are expected?

3. Is there a possible concern with drug interactions?

4. After 4 months of therapy, Jack experiences dizziness, dyspnea, and a rapid heart rate, and is taken to the emergency department. He is diagnosed with sustained PSVT, and intravenous verapamil does not help. What would the nurse think would be tried next?

Chapter 24

Antianginal Drugs

CHAPTER REVIEW

Choose the best answer for each of the following.

1. The purpose of antianginal drug therapy is which of the following?
   a. To increase myocardial oxygen demand
   b. To increase blood flow to peripheral arteries
   c. To increase blood flow to ischemic cardiac muscle
   d. To decrease blood flow to ischemic cardiac muscle

2. A patient taking nitroglycerin should be taught that a common adverse effect of this drug is which of the following?
   a. Blurred vision
   b. Dizziness
   c. Headache
   d. Weakness

3. Nitroglycerin is available in which of the following forms? Select all that apply.
   a. Continuous intravenous drip
   b. Intravenous bolus
   c. Sublingual spray
   d. Oral dosage forms
   e. Topical ointment
   f. Rectal suppository

4. For a patient using transdermal patches, the nurse recognizes that the best way to prevent tolerance to nitrates is to do which of the following?
   a. Leave the old patch on for 2 hours after applying a new patch.
   b. Apply a new patch every other day.
   c. Leave the patch off for 24 hours once a week.
   d. Remove the patch at night for 8 hours, and then apply a new patch in the morning.

5. Patients who are taking β-blockers for angina need to be taught which of the following about these drugs?
   a. They are for long-term prevention of angina episodes.
   b. They should be taken as soon as anginal pain occurs.
   c. Patients should discontinue if dizziness occurs.
   d. β-blockers should be carried with them at all times in case angina occurs.

6. Which type of antianginal medication is most effective for the treatment of coronary artery spasms?
   a. β-blockers
   b. Calcium channel blockers
   c. Nitrates
   d. Nitrites

CRITICAL THINKING AND APPLICATION

Answer the following questions on a separate sheet of paper.

7. The nurse is playing racquetball at a community centre when she notices a commotion at a gathering of senior citizens in a nearby room. She rushes in to find a man lying unconscious on the floor. Several people say that he is having a "heart attack." One man hands her a pill bottle and asks, "Would it help to give him one of my heart pills?" A woman agrees, saying, "Yes! Can't you put it under his tongue?" She see that the medication bottle is labelled Novo-Sorbide (isosorbide dinitrate). What does the nurse know about this medication, and what should she do?

8. Ms. Vickers is a 70-year-old woman seen in the emergency department for a laceration to her thumb. During her assessment, Ms. Vickers tells the nurse that she has been "tired and depressed" and has been having "nightmares" since her doctor prescribed heart medicine for her angina. Which drug does the nurse suspect Ms. Vickers is taking, and why?

9. During the nurse's home visit with Theresa, she shows him a journal entry describing the duration, time of onset, and severity of a recent angina attack. She reports no adverse effects to her nitroglycerin and shows him where she keeps the tablets, in a clear plastic pillbox on the kitchen windowsill. What does the nurse discuss with Theresa?

CASE STUDY

Read the scenario and answer the following questions on a separate sheet of paper.

While playing handball, 59-year-old Gideon experiences chest pain. He has had angina before and has sublingual nitroglycerin in his gym bag.

1. What type of angina is he experiencing?

2. What should he do to treat this episode of angina?

3. After he takes the nitroglycerin tablets, the chest pain did not subside. He wants his handball partner to drive him to the hospital. Is this what he should do at this time?

4. Other than nitroglycerin, which class of drugs is typically good for this type of angina?

Chapter 25
Antihypertensive Drugs

CRITICAL THINKING CROSSWORD

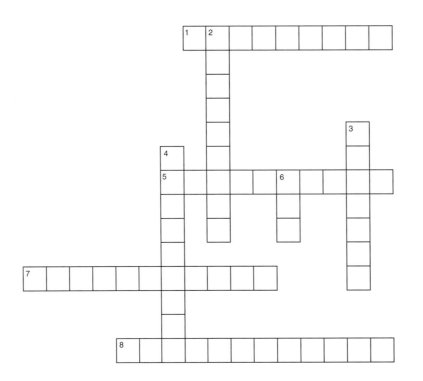

Across

1. High blood pressure associated with diseases such as renal, pulmonary, endocrine, and vascular diseases is known as _____ hypertension.
5. Another term for 3 Down.
7. A common adverse effect of adrenergic drugs involving a sudden drop in blood pressure when patients change position is known as _____ hypotension.
8. These drugs are used in the management of hypertensive emergencies.

Down

2. Another term for 3 Down.
3. Elevated systemic arterial pressure for which no cause can be found is known as _____ hypertension.
4. The primary effect of these drugs is to decrease plasma and extracellular fluid volumes.
6. Drugs that are often used as first-line drugs in the treatment of both heart failure and hypertension are known by the acronym _____ inhibitors.

CHAPTER REVIEW

Choose the best answer for each of the following.

1. Michael, age 46, has been taking clonidine HCl (Catapres) for 5 months. For the last 2 months, his blood pressure has been normal. During this office visit, he tells the nurse that he would like to stop taking the drug. The nurse's best response would be which of the following?
   a. "I'm sure the doctor will stop it—your blood pressure is normal now."
   b. "Your doctor will probably have you stop taking the drug for a month, and then we'll see how you do."
   c. "This drug should not be stopped suddenly; let's talk to your doctor."
   d. "It's likely that you can stop the drug if you exercise and avoid salty foods."

2. When administering angiotensin-converting enzyme (ACE) inhibitors, the nurse keeps in mind that adverse effects include which of the following? Select all that apply.
   a. Diarrhea
   b. Fatigue
   c. Restlessness
   d. Headaches
   e. A dry cough
   f. Tremors

3. A patient with type 2 diabetes mellitus has developed hypertension. The nurse knows that the blood pressure goal for this patient would be which of the following?
   a. Less than 110/80 mm Hg
   b. Less than 120/80 mm Hg
   c. Less than 130/80 mm Hg
   d. Less than 140/90 mm Hg

4. A patient is being treated for a hypertensive emergency. The nurse expects which drug to be used?
   a. sodium nitroprusside (Nipride)
   b. losartan potassium (Cozaar)
   c. captopril (Capoten)
   d. prazosin HCl (Minipress)

5. Julie, who is in her eighth month of pregnancy, has pre-eclampsia. Her blood pressure is 210/100 mm Hg this morning. This type of hypertension is classified as which of the following?
   a. Primary
   b. Idiopathic
   c. Essential
   d. Secondary

CRITICAL THINKING AND APPLICATION

Answer the following questions on a separate sheet of paper.

6. Mr. Quester, age 61, comes to the emergency department with symptoms of severe hypertensive emergency. The emergency department resident on call initiates therapy with sodium nitroprusside (Nipride). The patient is transferred to the intensive care unit and monitored. Hours later, his blood pressure falls to 100/60 mm Hg, and he is lethargic and complaining of feeling dizzy. What should the nurse do?

7. A patient has had an average blood pressure reading of 124/86 mm Hg for the last 3 months. He has a history of type 2 diabetes mellitus and had a myocardial infarction 6 months ago.
   a. Is this patient's hypertension considered normal? Explain your answer.
   b. Will drug therapy be ordered? Explain your answer.

8. Indicate which ACE inhibitor would be best for the following patients. Explain your answers.

   a. Irene, who has liver dysfunction, has high blood pressure and is seriously ill

   b. Kory, who has a history of poor adherence to his medication regimen

9. Mr. Bass will be starting prazosin HCl (Minipress) for hypertension. What should he be taught before he takes the first dose of this medication?

10. White and Black patients are known to react differently to antihypertensive agents.

    a. Which antihypertensives are considered more effective in white patients than in Black patients?

    b. Which antihypertensives are considered more effective in Black patients than in white patients?

CASE STUDY

Read the scenario and answer the following questions on a separate sheet of paper.

John, a 44-year-old man of African descent, has been seen twice in the last month for "blood pressure problems." At the first visit, his blood pressure was 144/90 mm Hg; at the second visit, his blood pressure was 154/96 mm Hg. The physician is preparing to start John on antihypertensive therapy.

1. What initial drug therapy would be appropriate for John? What factors are considered when choosing which drug to use?

2. If John also has a history of diabetes mellitus, what would be the blood pressure goal? Why?

3. John tells the nurse that he hopes this medication will not "slow him down" because he likes to "jump out of bed and get started" with his day. What teaching should the nurse provide for him to help him adjust to his blood pressure medication?

Chapter 26

Diuretic Drugs

CHAPTER REVIEW

Match each term with its corresponding definition.

1. _____ Diuretics

2. _____ Potassium-sparing diuretics

3. _____ Kaliuretic diuretics

4. _____ Osmotic diuretics

5. _____ Thiazides

6. _____ Ascites

7. _____ CAIs

8. _____ Loop diuretics

9. _____ Nephron

10. _____ Glomerular filtration rate

a. Potent diuretics that act along the ascending limb of the loop of Henle (furosemide [Lasix] is an example)

b. Abbreviation for the term that describes an index of how well the kidneys are functioning as filters

c. A general term for drugs that accelerate the rate of urine formation

d. The main structural unit of the kidney

e. A term for diuretics that cause the body to lose potassium

f. Diuretics that result in the diuresis of sodium and water and the retention of potassium (spironolactone [Aldactone] is an example)

g. Diuretics that act on the distal convoluted tubule, where they inhibit sodium and water resorption (hydrochlorothiazide [Apo-Hydro] is an example)

h. Abbreviation for a class of diuretics that inhibit the enzyme carbonic anhydrase; acetazolamide is an example

i. Drugs that induce diuresis by increasing the osmotic pressure of the glomerular filtrate, resulting in a rapid diuresis (mannitol is an example)

j. An abnormal intraperitoneal accumulation of fluid

Choose the best answer for each of the following.

11. Which of the following are indications for the use of diuretics? Select all that apply.
    a. To increase urine output
    b. To reduce uric acid levels
    c. To treat hypertension
    d. To treat open-angle glaucoma
    e. To treat edema associated with heart failure

12. When providing patient teaching to a patient who is taking a potassium-sparing diuretic such as spironolactone (Aldactone), the nurse should include which of the following?
    a. There are no dietary restrictions with this medication.
    b. The patient should consume foods high in potassium, such as bananas and orange juice.
    c. The patient should avoid foods high in potassium.
    d. The patient should drink 1 to 2 L of fluid per day.

13. When teaching a patient about diuretic therapy, the nurse notes that which of the following is the best time of day to take these medications?
    a. Morning
    b. Midday
    c. Bedtime
    d. Time of day does not matter

14. When monitoring a patient for hypokalemia related to diuretic use, the nurse looks for which possible symptoms?
    a. Nausea, vomiting, and anorexia
    b. Diarrhea and abdominal pain
    c. Orthostatic hypotension
    d. Muscle weakness and lethargy

15. A patient with severe heart failure has been started on therapy with a carbonic anhydrase inhibitor (CAI), but the nurse mentions that this medication may be stopped in a few days. Which of the following is the reason for this short treatment?
    a. CAIs are not the first choice for treatment of heart failure.
    b. CAIs lose their diuretic effect in 2 to 4 days because metabolic acidosis develops.
    c. It is expected that the CAIs will dramatically reduce the fluid overload related to the heart failure.
    d. Allergic reactions to the CAIs are common.

CRITICAL THINKING AND APPLICATION

Answer the following questions on a separate sheet of paper.

16. Ms. Andersen is a 62-year-old retired teacher who is being treated for diabetes and open-angle glaucoma. The physician has prescribed a diuretic as an adjunct drug in the management of Ms. Andersen's glaucoma.

    a. Which diuretic drug was probably prescribed?

    b. What undesirable effect of the drug does the physician need to consider?

17. The nurse is about to administer mannitol to Arthur, who is in early acute renal failure.

    a. What is the significance of Arthur's kidney blood flow and glomerular filtration in this situation?

    b. By what means does the nurse administer the mannitol? What special guidelines does she follow?

    c. Arthur later complains of a headache and chills. Should the mannitol therapy be ended? Explain your answer.

18. Mr. Ferrara has been admitted to the nurse's unit for treatment of ascites. He also has some kidney impairment and a history of heavy drinking.

   a. Which diuretic drug does the nurse expect will be administered to Mr. Ferrara?

   b. What monitoring will be performed frequently? Why?

19. Brendan, a 39-year-old bricklayer, is taking a thiazide for hypertension. During a follow-up visit, he tells the nurse that he thinks the drug is affecting his "love life."

   a. To what adverse effect of thiazide therapy is Brendan probably referring?

   b. While the nurse is talking to Brendan, she notices a package of licorice in Brendan's coat pocket. He tells her he eats the candy "for energy," especially because he has been feeling so tired the past couple of days. What does the nurse tell Brendan?

20. The nurse receives a call from Mrs. Hill, who recently started diuretic therapy for hypertension. Mrs. Hill is concerned because her neighbour, who also takes medication for hypertension, has told her not to eat a lot of bananas or other foods containing potassium. "But you told me to eat foods high in potassium," Mrs. Hill says, "What's going on?" What is the nurse's response to Mrs. Hill?

CASE STUDY

Read the scenario and answer the following questions on a separate sheet of paper.

Lily has been taking furosemide (Lasix) for 3 months as part of her treatment for heart failure. At this time, she is complaining that she is feeling tired and has muscle weakness and no appetite; her blood pressure is 100/50 mm Hg.

1. What do her symptoms suggest? How did this happen?

2. What dietary measures could she have taken to prevent this problem?

The physician switches her medication to spironolactone (Aldactone).

3. How does this drug differ from furosemide (Lasix)?

4. For what drug interactions should the nurse check before she begins taking spironolactone?

Chapter 27

Fluids and Electrolytes

CHAPTER REVIEW

Choose the best answer for each of the following.

1. Common uses of crystalloids include which of
   the following? Select all that apply.
   a. Fluid replacement
   b. Promotion of urinary flow
   c. Transport of oxygen to cells
   d. Replacement of electrolytes
   e. As maintenance fluids
   f. Replacement of clotting factors

2. The intravenous order for a newly admitted
   patient calls for "Normal saline to run at
   100 mL/hr." The nurse will choose which
   concentration of normal sodium?
   a. 0.33%
   b. 0.45%
   c. 0.9%
   d. 3.0%

3. A patient has been admitted with severe
   dehydration after working outside on a very
   hot day. The nurse expects which intravenous
   fluid to be ordered for rapid fluid replacement?
   a. Albumin
   b. Hetastarch
   c. Fresh frozen plasma
   d. 3% sodium chloride

4. When giving intravenous potassium, which of the
   following is important for the nurse to remember?
   a. Intravenous doses are preferred over oral
      dosage forms.
   b. Intravenous solutions should contain at
      least 50 mmol/L.
   c. Potassium must always be given in diluted
      form.
   d. Potassium should be given by slow intrave-
      nous bolus.

5. When a patient is receiving blood products,
   the nurse monitors for signs of a possible
   transfusion reaction, such as which of the
   following?
   a. Subnormal temperature and hypertension
   b. Apprehension, restlessness, fever, and chills
   c. Decreased pulse and respiration and fever
   d. Headache, nausea, and lethargy

6. Which product is used to increase clotting
   factor levels in patients with a demonstrated
   deficiency rather than for routine fluid
   resuscitation?
   a. Plasma protein fraction
   b. Fresh frozen plasma
   c. Packed red blood cells
   d. Albumin

CRITICAL THINKING AND APPLICATION

Answer the following questions on a separate sheet of paper.

7. List the advantages and disadvantages of using crystalloids to replace fluid in patients with dehydration.

8. Some fluids are known as *oxygen-carrying resuscitation fluids.*

   a. Which class of fluids is given this designation?

   b. Why are these fluids able to carry oxygen?

c. Why are they the most expensive of the three types of fluids, and why is their origin a potential problem for a recipient?

9. Tanya, a 16-year-old student, is brought to the clinic by her mother, who says that Tanya has been on "some sort of fad diet." The mother is concerned because Tanya is tired and weak. During her assessment, Tanya admits that she has been using laxatives and eating little during the past few weeks.

   a. What electrolyte imbalance is Tanya probably experiencing?

   b. Assuming that laboratory studies show the problem to be mild, how can it be corrected?

10. Mr. Sanchez, a 45-year-old postal carrier, has come to the emergency department sweating profusely and complaining of stomach cramps and diarrhea. He says that he has been "miserable" from the heat the past few days. His serum sodium level is 128 mmol/L.

    a. What electrolyte imbalance does the nurse suspect?

    b. The physician prescribes an oral medication and then asks the nurse to discuss dietary considerations with Mr. Sanchez. What does she tell Mr. Sanchez?

    c. What adverse effect of sodium may be of special concern for Mr. Sanchez?

11. Victor is receiving a transfusion of a blood product.

    a. The nurse observes Victor, knowing that an adverse reaction to the transfusion may be manifested by what signs and symptoms?

    b. Victor's wife is crying and says, "People get AIDS from transfusions. What happens if Victor gets AIDS?" What does the nurse tell her?

    c. The transfusion for Victor seems to be progressing smoothly. How often does the nurse check Victor's vital signs while he is receiving the transfusion?

    d. After 45 minutes, Victor is restless, and his pulse rate has increased. What does the nurse do?

CASE STUDY

Read the scenario and answer the following questions on a separate sheet of paper.

An older adult man is admitted to the unit with hypoproteinemia caused by chronic malnutrition. The nurse notes that he has some edema over his body, and his total protein level is 48 g/L.

1. What is the normal total protein level? What is the relationship between his serum total protein level and the edema the nurse has noted?

2. The nurse is preparing to give him one unit of 5% albumin. How does albumin work in this situation?

3. What advantages does albumin have over crystalloids in this situation?

4. For what adverse effects should the nurse monitor while he is receiving albumin?

Chapter 28

Coagulation Modifier Drugs

CHAPTER REVIEW

Match each definition with its corresponding term. (Note: Not all terms will be used.)

1. _____ A drug that prevents the lysis of fibrin, thereby promoting clot formation

2. _____ The termination of bleeding by mechanical or chemical means

3. _____ A substance that prevents platelet plugs from forming

4. _____ A drug that dissolves thrombi

5. _____ The general term for a substance that prevents or delays coagulation of the blood

6. _____ A laboratory test used to measure the effectiveness of heparin therapy

7. _____ A test used, along with another measure, to evaluate the effectiveness of warfarin sodium (Coumadin) therapy

8. _____ A standardized measure of the degree of coagulation achieved by drug therapy with warfarin sodium

9. _____ A substance that reverses the effect of heparin

10. _____ A substance that reverses the effect of warfarin sodium

11. _____ Naturally occurring tissue plasminogen activator secreted by vascular endothelial cells

12. _____ A blood clot that dislodges and travels through the bloodstream

a. Prothrombin time

b. Activated partial thromboplastin time (APTT)

c. International normalized ratio (INR)

d. streptokinase (Streptase)

e. alteplase (Activase)

f. Thrombus

g. Embolus

h. vitamin K

i. protamine sulfate

j. Antiplatelet drug

k. Antifibrinolytic

l. Thrombolytic drug

m. Anticoagulant

n. Hemostasis

Choose the best answer for each of the following.

13. For which of the following conditions is the use of anticoagulants appropriate? Select all that apply.
    a. Atrial fibrillation
    b. Thrombocytopenia
    c. Myocardial infarction
    d. Presence of mechanical heart valves
    e. Aneurysm
    f. Leukemia

14. During teaching of a patient who will be taking warfarin sodium (Coumadin) at home, which statement by the nurse is correct regarding over-the-counter drug use?
    a. "Choose nonsteroidal anti-inflammatory drugs as needed for pain relief."
    b. "Aspirin products may result in an increased anticoagulant effect."
    c. "Vitamin E therapy is recommended to improve the effect of warfarin sodium."
    d. "Mineral oil is the laxative of choice while taking anticoagulants."

15. Which drug has antiplatelet properties?
    a. acetylsalicytic acid (Aspirin)
    b. warfarin sodium (Coumadin)
    c. heparin sulfate (Heparin Leo)
    d. streptokinase (Streptase)

16. When administering subcutaneous heparin, the nurse should remember to do which of the following?
    a. Use the same sites for injection to reduce trauma.
    b. Use a 2.5 cm needle for subcutaneous injections.
    c. Inject the medication without aspirating for blood return.
    d. Massage the site after the injection to increase absorption.

17. During thrombolytic therapy, the nurse monitors for bleeding. Which symptoms may indicate a serious bleeding problem? Select all that apply.
    a. Hypertension
    b. Hypotension
    c. Decreased level of consciousness
    d. Increased pulse rate
    e. Restlessness

18. Which drug is indicated for the prevention and treatment of deep vein thrombosis after knee or hip replacement surgery?
    a. Antiplatelet drugs, such as acetylsalicytic acid (Aspirin)
    b. Adenosine diphosphate (ADP) inhibitors, such as clopidogrel (Plavix)
    c. Anticoagulants, such as warfarin sodium (Apo-Warfarin)
    d. Low-molecular-weight heparins, such as enoxaparin sodium (Lovenox)

CRITICAL THINKING AND APPLICATION

Answer the following questions on a separate sheet of paper.

19. Mrs. Walma, a 60-year-old homemaker, is receiving subcutaneous heparin therapy for the prevention of deep vein thrombosis. After the nurse gives Mrs. Walma her injection, she complains of pain and begins to rub the site. Is that a problem?

20. During cardiopulmonary bypass for heart surgery, Mr. Wong is intentionally given a large dose of heparin. The surgeon then determines that the effects of the heparin need to be reversed quickly.

    a. How will this be done?

    b. How will the amount of antidote be determined?

    c. What is the most commonly used test for determining the effects of heparin therapy?

21. Vitamin K is a reversal drug for warfarin sodium (Apo-Warfarin). How can its use cause a problem for a patient experiencing warfarin toxicity?

22. Following surgery, Mr. Thurman has a chest tube put in place. The site has been bleeding excessively. What type of drug might the physician prescribe in this situation, and why?

23. William, a 38-year-old writer who has von Willebrand's disease, has undergone emergency surgery after an automobile accident. What drug is used in the management of bleeding in patients such as William? What is its effect?

24. Tobias has been given alteplase (Activase) during treatment for acute myocardial infarction.

    a. Does the nurse expect Tobias to have an allergic reaction to the drug? Explain your answer.

    b. A few minutes later, Tobias suffers a reinfarction. What drug should Tobias receive now?

25. Ursula, an inpatient on the nurse's unit, is on anticoagulant therapy. The nurse enters her room to find that she is restless and confused.

    a. Why are these findings significant?

    b. In this case, what other problems might the nurse expect to find?

    c. What should the nurse do?

CASE STUDY

Read the scenario and answer the following questions on a separate sheet of paper.

After experiencing transient ischemic attacks (TIAs), Doug has been started on clopidogrel (Plavix). He has a history of atherosclerotic heart disease and has had problems with peptic ulcer disease.

1. He asks, "Why am I on this fancy medicine? Why can't I just take an Aspirin a day, like they say on television?" What does the nurse tell him?

2. What should Doug be taught to report to his health care provider while he is taking this drug?

3. What precautions should Doug follow while he is taking this drug?

4. What natural herbal products should be avoided while Doug is taking this drug?

Chapter 29

Antilipemic Drugs

CHAPTER REVIEW

Choose the best answer for each of the following.

1. Patients taking cholestyramine resin (Novo-Cholamine) may experience which of the following adverse effects?
   a. Blurred vision and photophobia
   b. Drowsiness and difficulty concentrating
   c. Diarrhea and abdominal cramps
   d. Belching and bloating

2. Dietary measures for the patient on antilipemic therapy include which of the following? Select all that apply.
   a. Taking supplements of fat-soluble vitamins
   b. Taking supplements of B vitamins
   c. Increasing fluid intake
   d. Choosing foods that are lower in cholesterol and saturated fats
   e. Increasing the intake of raw vegetables, fruit, and bran

3. In reviewing the history of a newly admitted cardiac patient, the nurse recognizes that which of the following conditions is a contraindication to the use of antilipemic therapy?
   a. Liver disease
   b. Kidney disease
   c. Coronary artery disease
   d. Diabetes mellitus

4. A woman is being screened in the cardiac clinic for risk factors for coronary artery disease. Which of the following would be considered a negative, or favourable, risk factor for her?
   a. High-density lipoprotein (HDL) cholesterol level of 0.77 mmol/L
   b. HDL cholesterol level of 1.9 mmol/L
   c. Early menopause
   d. Age of 57 years

5. A patient who has started taking nicotinic acid (Niacin) complains that he "hates the side effects." Which statement by the nurse is most appropriate?
   a. "You will soon build up tolerance to these side effects."
   b. "You should take the niacin on an empty stomach."
   c. "You can take the niacin every other day if the adverse effects are bothersome."
   d. "Try taking a small dose of ibuprofen (Motrin) or another nonsteroidal anti-inflammatory drug 30 minutes before taking the niacin."

6. Which lipoprotein is often called the "good cholesterol?"
   a. Very-low-density lipoprotein (VLDL)
   b. Low-density lipoprotein (LDL)
   c. High-density lipoprotein (HDL)
   d. Triglycerides

CRITICAL THINKING AND APPLICATION

Answer the following questions on a separate sheet of paper.

7. For each of the following drugs, name the antilipemic category and briefly describe how the drug lowers lipid levels.
   a. gemfibrozil (Lopid)
   b. nicotinic acid (niacin)
   c. lovastatin (Mevacor)
   d. cholestyramine resin (Novo-Cholamine)

8. Mr. Harris is a 46-year-old business executive who travels frequently. He is slightly overweight "from all that room service," but he did quit smoking 6 years ago. During a routine checkup, Mr. Harris is found to have an LDL cholesterol level of 6mmol/L. He says, "I'm a busy man! Just give me some pills. I've got a plane to catch!" Will the physician prescribe an antilipemic for Mr. Harris? Explain your answer.

9. Mr. Jahnke is a 49-year-old farmer. During assessment, the nurse discovers the following: Mr. Jahnke's mother is living, but his father "dropped dead of a heart attack" at 53 years of age. Mr. Jahnke is a smoker with mild asthma and some arthritis in his hands. His blood pressure today is 122/78 mm Hg, and laboratory studies show an HDL of 1.74 mmol/L. Discuss Mr. Jahnke's risk factors for high cholesterol.

10. Mrs. Kim has been treated with cholestyramine for type IIa hyperlipidemia for the past 2 months. She tells the nurse that she "can't stand being so irregular" and that she has developed another "embarrassing problem" as well. What is wrong with Mrs. Kim, and how can the nurse help her?

11. Justus is a 55-year-old attorney being treated with lovastatin (Mevacor) for hyperlipidemia. His current health status includes mild hypertension and a peptic ulcer. The nurse knows that nicotinic acid (niacin) is frequently prescribed as an adjunct to other antilipemic drugs. Would niacin be helpful for Justus? Explain your answer.

12. The nurse is visiting Mrs. Nguyen, a homebound patient who is being treated for hyperlipidemia and hypertension. During the visit, Mrs. Nguyen takes her antihypertensive medication and then begins stirring her dose of cholestyramine resin (Novo-Cholamine) into a glass of orange juice. What patient teaching does Mrs. Nguyen require?

CASE STUDY

Read the scenario and answer the following questions on a separate sheet of paper.

Mr. Miller has been diagnosed with type IIa hyperlipidemia and has been given a prescription for atorvastatin (Lipitor). He acts thrilled with the news and says, "Great! Now I don't have to worry about watching my diet because I'm on this medicine!"

1. Is he right? What type of dietary guidelines should Mr. Miller follow while on this therapy?

2. What therapeutic effects does the nurse hope to see as a result of his taking atorvastatin?

3. After 2 months of therapy, the nurse notes that Mr. Miller's liver enzymes are slightly elevated. Is this a concern, and what other laboratory work should be monitored while he is taking atorvastatin (Lipitor)?

4. Mr. Miller calls the office to complain about some muscle pain. He thought he had pulled a muscle during a tennis match, but the pain has not lessened in 3 days. Is this a concern?

Chapter 30

Pituitary Drugs

1. Complete the following table.

Hormone	Function	Mimicking Drug(s)
Adrenocorticotropic hormone (ACTH, corticotropin)	Targets adrenal gland; mediates adaptation to stressors; promotes synthesis of the following three hormones: **a.**	**b.**
Growth hormone	**c.**	**d.**
e.	Increases water resorption in the distal tubules and collecting duct of nephron; concentrates urine; potent vasoconstrictor	**f.**
Endogenous oxytocin	**g.**	**h.**

Choose the best answer for each of the following.

2. Cosyntropin is used for which of the following? Select all that apply.
   a. Treatment of diabetes insipidus
   b. Treatment of multiple sclerosis
   c. Stimulation of skeletal growth
   d. Prevention of carcinoid crisis
   e. Reduction of anti-inflammation
   f. Diagnosis of adrenocortical insufficiency

3. A nurse is administering octreotide (Sandostatin) to a patient who has a metastatic carcinoid tumour. The patient asks about the purpose of this drug. The nurse's best response would be which of the following?
   a. "This drug helps to reduce the size of your tumour."

   b. "This drug works to prevent the spread of your tumour."
   c. "Octreotide is given to reduce the nausea and vomiting you are having from the chemotherapy."
   d. "This drug helps to control the flushing and diarrhea that you are experiencing."

4. Which nursing diagnosis is most appropriate for a patient who is receiving a pituitary drug?
   a. Constipation
   b. Disturbed body image
   c. Impaired physical mobility
   d. Impaired skin integrity

5. The nurse should instruct a patient taking desmopressin acetate (DDAVP Spray) as a nasal spray for the treatment of diabetes insipidus to do which of the following to obtain maximum benefit from the drug?
   a. Clear the nasal passages after spraying the medication.
   b. Inhale the spray for full drug effect.
   c. If nasal congestion occurs, take an over-the-counter preparation to control mucus.
   d. Administer the nasal spray at the same time every day.

6. During assessment, the nurse discovers that a patient on corticotropin therapy is experiencing tremors and slight tetany. The nurse recognizes that these findings may indicate the development of which of the following?
   a. Hypokalemia
   b. Hyperkalemia
   c. Hypocalcemia
   d. Hypernatremia

CRITICAL THINKING AND APPLICATION

Answer the following questions on a separate sheet of paper.

7. Alexis has multiple sclerosis. She is experiencing pain associated with inflammation.

   a. What drug might the physician recommend for Alexis?

   b. For what cautions and contraindications should the nurse assess before this drug is administered?

   c. What else might the nurse include in assessing Alexis for treatment?

   d. Alexis is determined to be an appropriate candidate for this drug of choice. Draw up an appropriate patient teaching plan.

8. A nurse has recently begun working in a specialized endocrinology clinic. The nurse's first patient, Patricia, a grade 2 student, is not growing at the rate that is expected. The physician has determined that Patricia is a candidate for somatropin (Humatrope) therapy. Her parents are nervous about giving injections to Patricia. What should be emphasized when teaching her parents about giving this drug?

9. Jack, a 25-year-old man, has come to the clinic, asking for "growth hormone." He heard that a cousin, who was diagnosed with dwarfism, is taking the hormone to "get taller," and Jack wants to take this hormone, too. He is 154.4 cm tall. What does the nurse tell him?

CASE STUDY

Read the scenario and answer the following questions on a separate sheet of paper.

Mr. Collins has been experiencing severe thirst, which he reports, "of course makes me go to the bathroom all the time, it seems." He is also dehydrated despite the amounts of water he has been drinking.

1. Predict Mr. Collins's probable disorder and two likely drugs of choice for Mr. Collins.

2. How will the nurse assess Mr. Collins before administering these drugs?

3. As a result of the nurse's assessment, it has been determined that Mr. Collins should do well with desmopressin (DDAVP) therapy. Describe the treatment and its therapeutic effects (that is, how it mimics the natural hormone) on the patient.

4. Following the nurse's explanation, Mr. Collins says, "Okay, okay, but what does it do for me?" Explain the physical improvements Mr. Collins should be able to see.

Chapter 31

Thyroid and Antithyroid Drugs

CRITICAL THINKING CROSSWORD

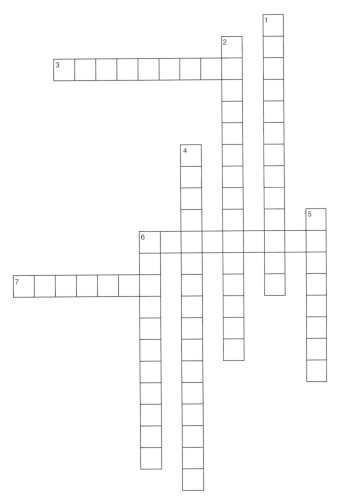

Across

3. The type of hypothyroidism that results from insufficient secretion of thyroid-stimulating hormone (TSH) from the pituitary gland.
6. The principal thyroid hormone that influences the metabolic rate.
7. The type of hypothyroidism that is due to the inability of the thyroid gland to perform a function.

Down

1. The most commonly prescribed synthetic thyroid hormone.
2. Excessive secretion of thyroid hormones.
4. A drug used to treat hyperthyroidism.
5. The type of hypothyroidism that stems from reduced secretion of thyrotropin-releasing hormone from the hypothalamus.
6. Another name for thyroid-stimulating hormone.

CHAPTER REVIEW

Choose the best answer for each of the following.

1. When should patients who begin therapy with levothyroxine (Eltroxin) expect effects from the medication?
   a. Immediately
   b. Within a few days
   c. Within a few weeks
   d. Within a few months

2. Mrs. Smith wants to switch brands of levothyroxine. The nurse's best response would be which of the following?
   a. "If you do this, you should reduce the dosage of your current brand before starting the new one."
   b. "Levothyroxine has been standardized, so there is only one brand."
   c. "It shouldn't matter if you switch brands; they are all very much the same."
   d. "You should check with your physician before switching brands."

3. Patient teaching for a patient taking antithyroid medication includes the need to avoid which foods?
   a. Soy products and seafood
   b. Bananas and oranges
   c. Dairy products
   d. Processed meats and cheese

4. Which of the following is a true statement that might be included in the nurse's teaching of patients taking thyroid medications? Select all that apply.
   a. Keeping a log or journal of individual responses and a graph of pulse rate, weight, and mood would be helpful.
   b. The medication should be discontinued if the adverse effects become too strong.
   c. The medication should be taken at the same time every day.
   d. Nervousness, irritability, and insomnia may be a result of a dosage that is too high.

5. Mr. Talbot is scheduled for a radioactive isotope study. Upon review of his medications, the scheduling nurse notes that he takes levothyroxine daily. Which statement is correct regarding the use of this medication before a radioactive isotope study?
   a. The patient should continue to take the medication as ordered.
   b. The patient should skip the medication on the morning of the test.
   c. The patient should stop the medication about 4 weeks before the test.
   d. The patient should reduce the dosage 1 week before the test.

CRITICAL THINKING AND APPLICATION

Answer the following questions on a separate sheet of paper.

6. Mrs. de Andrade, age 43, comes into the clinic complaining of hair loss, lethargy, and constipation. "I just can't eat anything," she says. As the nurse takes her blood pressure, the nurse notices that her skin feels thickened. She also seems to have a lump in her neck. Which of the disorders discussed in this chapter is Mrs. de Andrade most likely to have? Suggest several possible appropriate medications. Which of those is generally preferred? Why?

7. Ms. Hilton was diagnosed with Graves' disease 3 years ago. Today she reports symptoms of diarrhea, muscle weakness, fatigue, and palpitations. Also, she says, despite the diarrhea, she often has an increased appetite. She is also having trouble sleeping and wonders whether she is undergoing menopause because she suffers flushing, heat intolerance, and altered menstrual flow. As the nurse asks her questions about these symptoms, the nurse notes that she seems irritable. This is understandable, given her multiple symptoms; however, the nurse has known Ms. Hilton since she began treatment for

Graves' disease, and she has always been far from irritable, no matter how ill she felt. What does the nurse think is happening?

8. After undergoing a thyroidectomy as treatment for a thyroid tumour that turned out to be benign, Rebecca is given a prescription for levothyroxine (Eltroxin). "I thought I would be cured after this surgery!" she exclaims. "Why do I have to take a pill every day?" What does the nurse explain to Rebecca?

CASE STUDY

Read the scenario and answer the following questions on a separate sheet of paper.

Goldie, a 38-year-old teacher, has come to the clinic complaining of having "no energy or appetite," yet her weight has increased by 6.8 kg in the last month. The nurse notes that her hair is thin and her skin is dull. Laboratory work reveals an elevated level of thyroid-stimulating hormone.

1. What do Goldie's symptoms suggest? What medication does the nurse expect to be ordered for her?

2. Explain the concept of "euthyroid" as it would relate to Goldie's condition.

3. One month after therapy has begun, Goldie calls the office to complain that she "can't sleep at all" since she started taking the medication. She says she tries to take it at the same time every morning but often forgets and takes it at dinnertime. What teaching, if any, does she need to help her with this problem?

Chapter 32

Antidiabetic Drugs

CHAPTER REVIEW

Choose the best answer for each of the following.

1. When administering insulin, the nurse must keep in mind that the most immediate and serious adverse effect of insulin therapy is which of the following?
   a. Hyperglycemia
   b. Hypoglycemia
   c. Bradycardia
   d. Orthostatic hypotension

2. A dose of long-acting insulin has been ordered for bedtime for a diabetic patient. The nurse expects to give which type of insulin?
   a. Novolin ge Toronto
   b. insulin aspart (NovoRapid)
   c. Novilin ge NPH
   d. insulin glargine (Lantus)

3. Paulo is to be placed on an insulin drip to control his high blood glucose levels. Which type of insulin can be given intravenously?
   a. Novolin ge Toronto
   b. insulin aspart (NovoRapid)
   c. Novilin ge NPH
   d. insulin detemir (Levemir)

4. While monitoring a patient who is receiving insulin therapy, the nurse observes for signs of hypoglycemia, such as which of the following clusters of manifestations?
   a. Decreased pulse and respiratory rates and flushed skin
   b. Increased pulse rate and a fruity, acetone breath odour
   c. Weakness, sweating, and confusion
   d. Increased urine output and edema

5. When giving oral acarbose (Glucobay), the nurse should administer it at what time?
   a. 15 minutes before a meal
   b. 30 minutes before a meal
   c. With the first bite of a meal
   d. 1 hour after eating

6. A patient taking rosiglitazone (Avandia) tells the nurse, "There's my insulin pill!" The nurse describes the mechanism of action of rosiglitazone by explaining that this drug is not insulin, but works by which of the following mechanisms of action?
   a. It acts by stimulating the β cells of the pancreas to produce insulin.
   b. It acts by decreasing insulin resistance.
   c. It acts by inhibiting hepatic glucose production.
   d. It acts by decreasing intestinal absorption of glucose.

7. The sliding-scale insulin order reads: "Do bedside glucose testing before meals. For glucose results over 8.3 mmol/L, give regular (Humulin R) insulin, 1 unit for every 1.1 mmol/L over 8.3 mmol/L." If the blood glucose level is 13.2 mmol/L, the patient will receive _____ unit(s) of insulin.

CRITICAL THINKING AND APPLICATION

Answer the following questions on a separate sheet of paper.

8. Explain the mechanism of action of sitagliptin (Januvia).

9. Alice has mild hypoglycemia. Her physician has recommended dietary modifications to treat the condition.

   a. What general dietary guidelines should Alice follow?

   b. The nurse knows that one of the early signs of hypoglycemia is irritability. Why is this true?

   c. If Alice experiences hypoglycemia at home, what are the treatment options?

10. The nurse's co-worker, Bill, is in the medications room preparing a dose of Humulin-R to administer to a patient.

    a. Before he administers the medication, how should Bill verify the order?

    b. When the nurse enters the room, she notices that the insulin is cloudy. When she tells Bill to discard it, he says, "Insulin is supposed to look this way." Who is right?

    c. The nurse examines the vial. A date on the label indicates that it has been on the shelf in this room for 2 months. Is this a problem?

11. Alec, a 20-year-old university student, has been diagnosed with type 1 diabetes. The physician determines that Alec would be best treated with an insulin product that has an onset of 1 or 2 hours and a longer duration of 10–18 hours.

    a. What type of insulin does Alec require?

    b. What else might the physician need to consider when choosing a specific drug for Alec?

12. Mrs. Franklin, a 48-year-old homemaker, is 152.4 cm tall and weighs 81.6 kg. During a routine physical, laboratory studies indicate an elevated blood glucose level. The nurse's assessment of Mrs. Franklin reveals that she is a smoker with mild hypertension. The physician suspects type 2 diabetes.

    a. What initial treatment is indicated for Mrs. Franklin? Explain your answer.

    b. At a follow-up visit 3 months later, Mrs. Franklin's blood glucose level is still elevated. She has quit smoking, however, and has been walking for exercise. What treatment is indicated now?

13. Dennis is a 40-year-old taxicab dispatcher who takes chlorpropamide (Novo-Propamide). He comes to the emergency department late one Sunday evening complaining that he feels weak, vomited earlier, and has a headache, and that his face "feels hot." The nurse notes that Dennis has profound flushing and is sweating.

    a. What do Dennis's signs and symptoms indicate?

    b. What may have caused it? How can the nurse tell?

14. Natalia is taking insulin every morning, with sliding-scale coverage. The specified dosages are NPH (Novolin ge NPH) insulin, 20 units, every morning before breakfast; and regular (Novolin ge Toronto) insulin, sliding-scale coverage, before meals and at bedtime, as follows:

Blood glucose less than 11.1 mmol/L: no additional coverage
Blood glucose 11.1 to 13.8 mmol/L: 2 units regular insulin
Blood glucose 13.9 to 16.6 mmol/L: 4 units regular insulin
Blood glucose more than 16.7 mmol/L: 6 units regular insulin
Blood glucose more than 19.4 mmol/L: call for orders

How much insulin will Natalia receive in the following circumstances?

a. Before breakfast, if her blood glucose level is 15.3 mmol/L
b. Before lunch, if her blood glucose level is 10.9 mmol/L
c. Before dinner, if her blood glucose level is 18.2 mmol/L

CASE STUDY

Read the scenario and answer the following questions on a separate sheet of paper.

The physician is planning to prescribe gliclazide (Diamicron) for Mr. Dressel, a 50-year-old financial advisor with a history of renal failure. In particular, Mr. Dressel requires treatment for the short-term elevation in his blood glucose level that occurs after he eats.

1. Why did the physician choose a second-generation sulfonylurea rather than, for example, chlorpropamide (Novo-Propamide)?

2. Why would gliclazide be a good choice for Mr. Dressel?

3. When should he take this drug?

4. A few weeks later, Mr. Dressel develops influenza. He is vomiting and has been unable to eat all day. What should he do, and why?

Chapter 33

Adrenal Drugs

CHAPTER REVIEW

Choose the best answer for each of the following.

1. Jonathan has been taking prednisone (Winpred) following a severe reaction to poison ivy. He notices that the dosage of the medication decreases; he asks the nurse why he must continue the medication and why he cannot just stop taking it now that the skin rash is better. The nurse knows that which of the following is the best response?
   a. Sudden discontinuation of this medication may cause an adrenal crisis.
   b. Jonathan would experience withdrawal symptoms if the drug were discontinued abruptly.
   c. Cushing's syndrome may develop as a reaction to a sudden drop of serum cortisone levels.
   d. Jonathan can stop taking the medication if his rash is better.

2. Which medication is the preferred oral glucocorticoid for anti-inflammatory or immunosuppressant purposes?
   a. fludrocortisone (Florinef)
   b. dexamethasone (Dexasone)
   c. prednisone (Winpred)
   d. hydrocortisone (Cortef)

3. When monitoring a patient who is taking corticosteroids, the nurse observes for adverse effects, including which of the following? Select all that apply.
   a. Fragile skin
   b. Increased glucose levels
   c. Nervousness
   d. Hypotension
   e. Weight loss
   f. Drowsiness

4. A patient has Cushing's syndrome. The nurse expects which drug to be used to inhibit the function of the adrenal cortex?
   a. dexamethasone (Dexasone)
   b. prednisone (Winpred)
   c. hydrocortisone (Cortef)
   d. fludrocortisone (Florinef)

5. A patient who has been taking corticosteroids has developed a "moon face" and facial redness, and has many bruises on her arms. The most appropriate nursing diagnosis would be which of the following?
   a. Risk for infection
   b. Imbalanced nutrition (less than body requirements)
   c. Deficient fluid volume
   d. Disturbed body image

6. Because corticosteroids may cause sodium retention, the nurse should closely monitor patients with which condition when administering corticosteroids?
   a. Diabetes mellitus
   b. Seizure disorders
   c. Heart failure
   d. Hyperthyroidism

CRITICAL THINKING AND APPLICATION

Answer the following questions on a separate sheet of paper.

7. Ms. Rivera, a 30-year-old hospital receptionist, is receiving glucocorticoid therapy following a kidney transplant. The nurse is reviewing her drug regimen with her when she mentions that she frequently uses acetylsalicytic acid (Aspirin) or ibuprofen (Motrin) to treat problems such as headaches or menstrual cramps. She also says that she enjoys walking for exercise and likes to visit sick children on the hospital's pediatric ward when she has time. What issues does the nurse discuss with Ms. Rivera?

8. Peter, a 21-year-old mechanic, has developed a severe skin rash after a camping trip. The physician is planning to prescribe prednisone. The nursing assessment reveals that Peter has type 1 diabetes.

    a. Does that finding affect Peter's treatment? Explain your answer.

    b. To help minimize gastrointestinal effects, what suggestions would the nurse have for someone taking an oral form of the systemic adrenal drugs?

9. The nurse is watching a student nurse prepare to apply a topical glucocorticoid to a patient's skin rash. After putting on gloves, she places some of the medication on her finger. Should the nurse intervene, or is the student nurse doing fine so far? What other consideration is involved in determining the technique for applying a topical drug?

10. Nina has been prescribed a steroid drug delivered via inhaler. What special instructions does the nurse give her?

CASE STUDY

Read the scenario and answer the following questions on a separate sheet of paper.

Cheri is in the urgent care centre because of an exacerbation of asthma. She is usually able to control it with inhaled bronchodilators, but the physician decides to give her a short course of prednisone in a dose that starts high and then tapers down over a week's time.

1. Why is the dose tapered instead of just discontinued after a week?

2. What are potential effects of long-term therapy?

3. Is this drug a glucocorticoid or a mineralocorticoid? Explain the difference.

4. What time of day should Cheri take this drug? Explain.

Chapter 34

Women's Health Drugs

CHAPTER REVIEW

Choose the best answer for each of the following.

1. When reviewing the health history of a patient who wants to begin taking oral contraceptives, the nurse recalls that contraindications include which of the following? Select all that apply.
   a. Multiple sclerosis
   b. Pregnancy
   c. Thromboembolic disorders
   d. Breast cancer
   e. Abnormal vaginal bleeding

2. When teaching patients about postmenopausal estrogen replacement therapy, which statement is correct?
   a. "The smallest dose that is effective will be prescribed."
   b. "Oral forms should be taken on an empty stomach for best absorption."
   c. "Estrogen therapy should be long term to prevent menopausal symptoms."
   d. "If estrogen is taken, supplemental calcium will not be needed."

3. When combination oral contraceptives are used to provide postcoital emergency contraception, the nurse should remember which of the following facts?
   a. They are not effective if the woman is already pregnant.
   b. They should be taken within 12 hours of unprotected intercourse.
   c. They are given in one dose.
   d. They are intended to terminate pregnancy.

4. When reviewing an order for dinoprostone (Prostin E2) cervical gel, the nurse recalls that this drug is used for which of the following purposes ?
   a. To induce abortion during the third trimester.
   b. To improve cervical inducibility ("ripening") near term for labour induction.
   c. To soften the cervix in women who are experiencing infertility problems.
   d. To reduce postpartum uterine atony and hemorrhage.

5. When is the occurrence of spontaneous labour more commonly considered a spontaneous abortion or miscarriage?
   a. At any time during the pregnancy
   b. Before the 20th week
   c. Between the 20th and 37th weeks
   d. After the 37th week

6. What patient teaching is appropriate for the patient taking alendronate (Fosamax)? Select all that apply.
   a. Take on an empty stomach.
   b. Take at night just before going to bed.
   c. Take with an 8 oz glass of water.
   d. Take with a sip of water.
   e. Take first thing in the morning upon arising.
   f. Do not lie down for at least 30 minutes after taking.

CRITICAL THINKING AND APPLICATION

Answer the following questions on a separate sheet of paper.

7. Isabelle is a 48-year-old woman exhibiting symptoms of menopause. Assessment of Isabelle reveals a history of depression and mild arthritis.

   a. What does the nurse need to ask Isabelle, and why?

b. The physician decides to prescribe estrogen therapy. At this time, what does the nurse know about the dose and the length of time the estrogen will be administered?

8. Ms. Boutrimas is a 25-year-old paralegal diagnosed with diabetes. She is at the physician's office today because her menstrual periods have ceased. The physician has decided to prescribe a hormonal drug.

a. Which drug will the physician likely prescribe?

b. What adjustments to Ms. Boutrimas's existing drug regimen might need to be made?

9. Jacklyn receives a prescription for combined norethindrone/ethinylestradiol (Estalis) for birth control purposes. At a follow-up visit 4 months later, she tells the nurse, "I am really messing up. I take the pills for 3 weeks, but when I'm off them for a week, sometimes I don't remember to start again!"

a. What might the nurse suggest to help Jacklyn?

b. Jacklyn then expresses concern that her menstrual bleeding, now that she is on birth control pills, is "nothing compared with what it used to be." She asks whether she is okay. What does the nurse tell Jacklyn?

10. Ms. Stephanopoulos, a sales associate in a bookstore, is being treated for fertility problems. She is currently on a drug regimen that includes chorionic gonadotropin (Pregnyl) and menotropins (Menopur).

a. Why is Ms. Stephanopoulos taking two fertility drugs?

b. After the first course of treatment, Ms. Stephanopoulos does not become pregnant. Describe her next course of treatment.

11. Mrs. Ingalls has been taking estrogen therapy for several weeks. During a routine checkup, she sheepishly tells the nurse that she has not been able to quit smoking yet. She also mentions that she is going to Aruba for a vacation next month. What patient teaching does Mrs. Ingalls require?

12. Mrs. Vu, age 33 years, comes in for her yearly gynecological examination, and the physician recommends alendronate (Fosamax), 5 mg daily. Mrs. Vu experienced early menopause last year and asks the nurse, "Why did the doctor wait until now to start me on estrogen? I didn't need it before."

a. What does the nurse explain about the purpose of this medication?

b. What risk factors might Mrs. Vu have to support therapy with alendronate?

CASE STUDY

Read the scenario and answer the following questions on a separate sheet of paper.

Ms. O'Hara, a 34-year-old computer programmer, is having mild contractions. She is in the thirtieth week of gestation, and the physician determines that she is experiencing premature labour.

1. What nonpharmacological treatment is the physician likely to prescribe?

2. In Canada, are there other strategies that may be used to delay preterm labour?

Chapter 35

Men's Health Drugs

CHAPTER REVIEW

Choose the best answer for each of the following.

1. Jack, a member of the university hockey team, asks his friend's mother, who is a nurse, about taking steroids to help him "beef up" his muscles. Which of the following is true?
   a. There should be no problems as long as he does not exceed the recommended dose.
   b. Long-term use may cause a life-threatening liver condition.
   c. He would need to be careful to watch for excessive weight loss.
   d. These drugs also tend to increase sperm count.

2. In which of the following situations would androgens be prescribed for a woman? Select all that apply.
   a. Development of secondary sex characteristics
   b. Fibrocystic breast disease
   c. Ovarian cancer
   d. Treatment of endometriosis
   e. Postmenopausal osteoporosis prevention
   f. Metastatic breast cancer

3. Samuel will be receiving testosterone therapy for male hypogonadism and has a new prescription for transdermal testosterone (Androderm) patches. The nurse needs to include which teaching about the use of this medication?
   a. The patch should be applied only on the scrotum.
   b. The patch should not be applied on the scrotum.
   c. If the adverse effects become bothersome, the patient should stop using the patch.
   d. The patch should be applied to a different area of the upper body each day.

4. Before a patient begins therapy with finasteride (Proscar), the nurse should make sure that which laboratory test has been performed?
   a. Blood glucose level
   b. Complete blood count
   c. Urinalysis
   d. Prostate-specific antigen (PSA) level

5. Mr. Hu is taking finasteride (Proscar) for the treatment of benign prostatic hypertrophy. His wife, who is 3 months pregnant, is worried about the adverse effects that may occur with this drug. Which statement by the nurse is the most important at this time?
   a. "Gastric upset may be reduced if he takes this drug on an empty stomach."
   b. "You should notice therapeutic effects of increased libido and erection within 1 month."
   c. "This medication should not be handled by pregnant women because it may harm the fetus."
   d. "You may experience transient hair loss while taking this medication."

6. Which drug is used, in low doses, for androgenic alopecia in both men and women?
   a. finasteride (Propecia)
   b. nandrolone (Deca Durabolin)
   c. danazol (Cyclomen)
   d. minoxidil (Rogaine)

CRITICAL THINKING AND APPLICATION

Answer the following questions on a separate sheet of paper.

7. Mr. Michaels is being treated for hypogonadism. He has been taking intramuscular injections of testosterone cypionate. Today he will be switched to an oral dosage form, testosterone undeconate (Andriol).

    a. Mr. Michaels is skeptical of switching drugs and asks for more information. Explain specifically why oral testosterone does not often work well and why oral testosterone undeconate (Andriol) capsules will be effective.

    b. Discuss potential contraindications that might apply to this patient.

8. Mr. Koo, a recent immigrant to Canada, is living temporarily with his sister and her two small children. He has been diagnosed with male hypogonadism and has been prescribed testosterone in the AndroGel pump form. AndroGel comes as a 60 actuation metered-dose pump.

    a. English is a second language for Mr. Koo. Describe to him what "60 actuation metered-dose" means and what its implications are in terms of drug dosing.

    b. What specific instructions should Mr. Koo receive about the use of the pump?

9. Mr. Olafson has been prescribed finasteride (Proscar) for benign prostatic hypertrophy. He asks, "How does it work?" The nurse explains that it will cause his prostate to decrease in size and will alleviate discomfort. "No," he says. "You don't understand. I'm not a pharmacist, but I am a chemist. Tell me how it works."

    a. Tell him everything you know about how finasteride works.

    b. What are the most important things to include in his patient teaching plan?

10. Explain the application method for the testosterone (Androderm) patch.

CASE STUDY

Read the scenario and answer the following questions on a separate sheet of paper.

Mr. Ang, age 72, has asked the doctor for "help with a private matter." He tells the physician that he would like to try "that drug that helps with a certain problem."

1. What assessment findings may contraindicate the use of sildenafil in Mr. Ang?

2. If Mr. Ang is a candidate for therapy with sildenafil citrate (Viagra), what patient teaching should he receive?

3. What concerns would there be about his liver function? About his vision?

4. When should he take this medication?

Chapter 36

Antihistamines, Decongestants, Antitussives, and Expectorants

CHAPTER REVIEW

Choose the best answer for each of the following.

1. Which of the following are correct statements to include in patient teaching about antihistamine use? Select all that apply.
   a. Antihistamines are best tolerated when taken with meals.
   b. The patient can suck on hard candy or chew gum if dry mouth is experienced.
   c. The main adverse effect of antihistamines is drowsiness.
   d. Over-the-counter medications are generally safe to use with antihistamines.

2. A patient asks the nurse for advice about one of the newer antihistamines that does not cause drowsiness. Which of the following drugs is appropriate?
   a. desloratadine (Aerius)
   b. diphenhydramine HCl (Aller-Aide)
   c. dimenhydrinate (Gravol)
   d. meclizine HCl (Bonamine)

3. Which drugs are considered first-line drugs for the treatment of nasal congestion?
   a. Antihistamines such as diphenhydramine HCl
   b. Decongestants such as oxymetazoline (Vicks Sinex)
   c. Antitussives such as dextromethorphan (Benylin)
   d. Expectorants such as guaifenesin (Robitussin Liquid)

4. When giving an antitussive, the nurse remembers that they are used primarily to do which of the following?
   a. To relieve nasal congestion
   b. To thin secretions to ease the removal of excessive secretions
   c. To stop the cough reflex when the cough is nonproductive
   d. To suppress productive and nonproductive coughs

5. Which teaching is appropriate for the patient receiving an expectorant?
   a. Avoid fluids for 30 to 35 minutes after the dose.
   b. Drink plenty of fluids, unless contraindicated, to aid in expectoration of sputum.
   c. Avoid driving or operating heavy machinery while taking this medication.
   d. Patients should expect their secretions to become thicker.

6. A patient has been self-medicating with diphenhydramine to help her sleep. She calls the clinic nurse to ask, "Why do I feel so tired during the day after I take this pill? I get a good night's sleep!" Which statement by the nurse is correct?
   a. "You are probably getting too much sleep."
   b. "You are taking too much of the drug."
   c. "This drug is not really meant to help people sleep."
   d. "This drug often causes a 'hangover effect' during the day after taking it."

CRITICAL THINKING AND APPLICATION

Answer the following questions on a separate sheet of paper.

7. Why are histamine-1 (H$_1$) blockers most beneficial when given early in a histamine-mediated reaction?

8. Do the traditional antihistamines have any advantages over the newer, nonsedating antihistamines? Explain your answer.

9. Mrs. Ling was seen in the office several days ago with a common cold. She has been on decongestant therapy with oxymetazoline HCl (Afrin Sinus and Allergy) since that time. Today she calls to say, "I thought I was getting over this, but suddenly my nose is more stuffed up than ever." Does Mrs. Ling possibly need a stronger dosage of decongestant? Explain your answer.

10. Keith has been using a topical nasal decongestant for the past few days. He calls the physician's office to report that he is feeling nervous and dizzy and that his heart seems to be racing. What might be the cause of Keith's symptoms?

11. How does dextromethorphan (Benylin) differ from other antitussive drugs in its mechanism of action? What about its drug interaction profile?

12. One day the nurse encounters his neighbour, Irene, as he is returning home from work. She is on her way to the drugstore, she tells him, because she has been experiencing a nonproductive cough and wants to get "a cough medicine to loosen things up." The nurse recalls Irene mentioning a few months ago that she has problems with her thyroid. Does he wish Irene good luck and continue on his way? Explain your answer.

13. Lisa is a 5-year-old patient who has bronchitis accompanied by a nonproductive cough. The physician has prescribed guaifenesin (Robitussin Liquid) for the cough. Lisa's father tells the nurse that his 11-year-old son was prescribed Robitussin A-C several months ago for a severe cough. He asks whether his son's cough medicine would help Lisa, since "there is plenty left in the bottle." What does the nurse tell him?

14. Justin calls the nurse at the office because he experiences "palpitations and a racing heart" every morning after breakfast. Upon questioning, he states that he has been taking a decongestant for a cold and has been drinking an extra cup of coffee in the morning "to get going" since the cold has kept him from sleeping well. What could be his problem?

CASE STUDY

Read the scenario and answer the following questions on a separate sheet of paper.

James, a 35-year-old electrician, is seen in the emergency department with a rash on his arms and hands that appeared after he was working in his yard. The nurse suspects that the physician will prescribe topical diphenhydramine (Anti-Itch Cream), but during the nursing assessment, James says that he has diabetes.

1. How does James's diagnosis of diabetes affect his possible treatment with diphenhydramine?

2. If James does receive a topical diphenhydramine, what other drug might be found in combination with it?

The topical medication did not help his rash, and James has been switched to oral diphenhydramine. He tells the nurse that he expects to return to work tomorrow and hopes this medication "does the trick."

3. What cautions, if any, should James be aware of while taking this medication?

4. Are there any concerns with drug interactions?

Chapter 37

Bronchodilators and Other Respiratory Drugs

CHAPTER REVIEW

Choose the best answer for each of the following.

1. Frequent use of bronchodilators may cause which adverse effects? Select all that apply.
   a. Blurred vision
   b. Increased heart rate
   c. Decreased heart rate
   d. Nausea
   e. Nervousness
   f. Tremors

2. Maggie is taking a leukotriene antagonist. The nurse should include which of the following when teaching Maggie about this class of drugs?
   a. If a dose is missed, Maggie may take a double dose to maintain therapeutic blood levels.
   b. Maggie should gargle or rinse her mouth after taking the medication.
   c. The medication should should be taken at the first sign of bronchospasm.
   d. She should administer the medication consistently and be aware that improvement should be seen within 1 week of use.

3. Which drug acts by blocking leukotrienes, thus reducing inflammation in the lungs?
   a. salbutamol sulfate (Airomir)
   b. cromolyn sodium (Nalcrom)
   c. theophylline (Theolair)
   d. montelukast (Singulair)

4. A patient in status asthmaticus has not yet responded to epinephrine. The nurse will expect which of the following drugs to be used next?
   a. salbutamol sulfate (Ventolin)
   b. aminophylline
   c. theophylline (Theolair)
   d. montelukast (Singular)

5. When a patient is taking parenteral xanthine derivatives, such as aminophylline, the nurse should monitor for which adverse effect?
   a. Decreased respirations
   b. Hypotension
   c. Tachycardia
   d. Hypoglycemia

6. A patient who is taking a β-adrenergic agonist for bronchodilation may also take which type of inhaled drug for its anti-inflammatory effects?
   a. Corticosteroid
   b. Anticholinergic
   c. Xanthine derivative
   d. Antileukotriene

CRITICAL THINKING AND APPLICATION

Answer the following questions on a separate sheet of paper.

7. What are the three main etiological factors of asthma, and their causes?

8. Tom, a 70-year-old retiree who smoked for 40 years, has been diagnosed with chronic obstructive pulmonary disease (COPD); the treatment regimen prescribed includes theophylline (Theolair). After a few weeks, Tom tells the nurse that he is experiencing nausea and "bad heartburn at night." The laboratory studies show the level of theophylline in his blood to be 130 micromoles/L. What might be wrong with Tom, and how can it be corrected?

9. Willie is a 9-year-old boy who is brought to the emergency department by his aunt because he is having an acute asthma attack. The physician orders epinephrine subcutaneously. How does the nurse calculate the dosage for Willie?

10. Sylvia has come to the clinic today complaining of nausea, palpitations, and anxiety. She says that her heart feels "as if it's going to fly out of my chest." Physical examination confirms an increased heart rate. Sylvia's records indicate that she has asthma, for which she uses a salbutamol (Ventolin) inhaler. What does the nurse suspect might be wrong with Sylvia, and what suggestions does the nurse have for her?

11. Mrs. Di Risio, a 65-year-old office manager, has arthritis, glaucoma, and emphysema. The physician is planning prophylactic treatment for her emphysema.

    a. What three types of drugs might be considered for a patient with COPD?

    b. What factor must the physician keep in mind when determining the best drug for Mrs. Di Risio?

12. Several months ago, the physician prescribed an orally administered corticosteroid for Mr. Zoller, who has chronic bronchial asthma.

    a. What are the disadvantages of administering the corticosteroids orally?

    b. Today the physician adds beclomethasone dipropionate (QVAR) to Mr. Zoller's drug regimen and also reduces the dosage of the oral corticosteroid. Is that safe?

13. Sam is a 10-year-old girl who is to be treated with Advair for asthma.

    a. What drugs are contained in Advair? Explain why they would be used in Sam's case.

    b. What other drug would be an important component of Sam's daily routine? Explain.

CASE STUDY

Read the scenario and answer the following questions on a separate sheet of paper.

Jennie has been treated for adult-onset asthma for 3 years. Today she has started taking montelukast (Singular), one 10-mg tablet daily.

1. How does this medication differ from traditional antiasthma drugs?

2. Jennie says, "I hope this medicine works better than the other one I took when I had an asthma attack." What should the nurse's reply be?

3. Jennie takes ibuprofen (Advil) on occasion for arthritic pain. What should the nurse advise about taking this medication with montelukast?

4. After 3 months, Jennie stops taking the montelukast. She says that her symptoms are "better, and I don't want to take medicine unless I need it." Is this appropriate?

Chapter 38

Antibiotics Part 1: Sulfonamides, Penicillins, Cephalosporins, Macrolides, and Tetracyclines

CRITICAL THINKING CROSSWORD

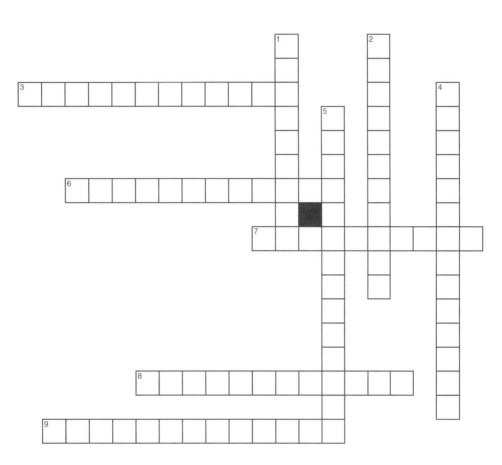

Across

3. Antibiotics taken before exposure to an infectious organism in an effort to prevent the development of infection.
6. The classification for the drug doxycycline (Doxycin).
7. An antibiotic derived from a fungus or mould often seen on bread or fruit.
8. Antibiotics that kill bacteria.
9. The classification for the drug cefazolin.

Down

1. The classification for the drug erythromycin (Apo-Erythro E-C).
2. The classification for the drug sulfisoxazole.
4. Antibiotics that inhibit the growth of bacteria.
5. An infection that occurs during antimicrobial treatment for another infection and involves overgrowth of a nonsusceptible organism.

CHAPTER REVIEW

Choose the best answer for each of the following.

1. A drug interaction occurs with penicillins and which of the following? Select all that apply.
   a. Alcohol
   b. Oral contraceptives
   c. digoxin (Lanoxin)
   d. Nonsteroidal anti-inflammatory drugs
   e. warfarin (Coumadin)
   f. Anticonvulsants

2. Which intervention is important for the nurse to perform before beginning antibiotic therapy?
   a. Obtain a specimen for culture and sensitivity.
   b. Give with an antacid to reduce gastrointestinal upset.
   c. Monitor for adverse effects.
   d. Restrict oral fluids.

3. Which of the following teaching points will the nurse include in patient teaching about a tetra-cycline antibiotic?
   a. Take it with milk.
   b. Take it with 240 mL of water.
   c. Take it 30 minutes before taking iron preparations.
   d. Use an antacid to decrease gastrointestinal discomfort.

4. A patient is to receive antibiotic therapy with a cephalosporin. When assessing the patient's drug history, the nurse recognizes that an allergy to which type of drug may be a possible contraindication to cephalosporin therapy?
   a. Cardiac glycosides
   b. Thiazide diuretics
   c. Penicillins
   d. Macrolides

5. When asked about drug allergies, a patient says, "I can't take sulfa drugs because I'm allergic to them." Which question should the nurse ask next?
   a. "Do you have any other drug allergies?"
   b. "Who prescribed the drug for you?"
   c. "How long ago did this happen?"
   d. "What happened when you took the sulfa drug?"

6. A patient is being prepared for colon surgery, and will be receiving cefazolin 1 g intravenously before surgery. He asks the nurse why he needs to take this drug before surgery. Which of the following is the nurse's best response?
   a. "This drug helps to clear out your bowels before surgery."
   b. "This drug helps to reduce the number of bacteria in your intestines before surgery."
   c. "This drug is given to sterilize your bowel before surgery."
   d. "This drug is given to prevent an infection after surgery."

CRITICAL THINKING AND APPLICATION

Answer the following questions on a separate sheet of paper.

7. Mr. Renville, a 50-year-old banker, is scheduled for colorectal surgery tomorrow. The surgeon is planning to administer a prophylactic antibiotic. What drug is frequently used for this purpose, and why?

8. Sean is a 19-year-old first-year university student who has been diagnosed with gonorrhea. The physician has prescribed doxycycline (Doxycin) therapy. During the nursing assessment, the nurse and Sean discuss his diet, which includes "lots of meat, milk, and veggies." Sean also says that he jogs frequently and is a member of the tennis team.

   a. In addition to instruction about sexually transmitted diseases, what patient teaching does Sean require?

   b. A few days later, Sean calls and complains of an upset stomach and diarrhea. What does the nurse suspect might be the problem Sean is experiencing?

9. Sandra, a 59-year-old homemaker, has bronchitis and has been taking an antibiotic for 1 week. She calls the nurse and complains of severe itching and a whitish discharge in her vaginal area. What has happened, and what caused it?

CASE STUDY

Read the scenario and answer the following questions on a separate sheet of paper.

A 78-year-old patient, admitted to the hospital with a stroke 2 days earlier, has developed a urinary tract infection. His Foley catheter is draining urine that is cloudy and dark yellowish-orange, with a strong odour. Strands of pus are also visible in the urine. He is receiving an intravenous heparin infusion and has a history of type 2 diabetes. The physician orders combination sulfamethoxazole trimethoprim (Protrin).

1. What should be assessed before giving this medication?

2. Are there any potential drug interactions?

3. Why was this particular antibiotic chosen?

4. Is this antibiotic bactericidal or bacteriostatic? Explain.

Chapter 39

Antibiotics Part 2: Aminoglycosides, Fluoroquinolones, and Other Drugs

CHAPTER REVIEW

Choose the best answer for each of the following.

1. When patients are receiving aminoglycosides, the nurse must monitor for tinnitus, which may indicate which of the following?
   a. Cardiotoxicity
   b. Hepatotoxicity
   c. Ototoxicity
   d. Nephrotoxicity

2. A patient has been admitted to the unit with a stage IV pressure ulcer. After 2 days, the wound culture comes back positive for methicillin-resistant *Staphylococcus aureus* (MRSA). The nurse knows that the drug of choice for the treatment of MRSA infection is which of the following?
   a. vancomycin (Vancocin)
   b. gentamicin sulfate
   c. ciprofloxacin (Cipro)
   d. dapsone

3. For which of the following effects should a patient who is receiving vancomycin therapy notify the nurse immediately? Select all that apply.
   a. Ringing in the ears
   b. Dizziness
   c. Hearing loss
   d. Fullness in the ears

4. Metronidazole (Flagyl) is an effective antimicrobial used in the management of which of the following disorders?
   a. *Clostridium difficle*
   b. Methicillin-resistant *S. aureus*
   c. *Mycobacterium leprae*
   d. *Chlamydia*

CRITICAL THINKING AND APPLICATION

Answer the following questions on a separate sheet of paper.

5. Angie has a severe infection and is receiving an aminoglycoside once a day. She says, "They tell me I have a terrible infection. Why am I not getting the antibiotic more than once a day? I don't understand!" What should the nurse tell her?

6. Explain the concept of "trough" levels during aminoglycoside therapy and the way in which kidney function is monitored.

7. Greg has been taking amiodarone (Cordarone) for a heart rhythm problem. He has developed an infection from an open wound, and the sensitivity report indicates that levofloxacin is the best choice to fight this infection. Are there any concerns?

8. Nitrofurantoin (Macrodantin) has been ordered for a patient who has a severe urinary tract infection caused by *Escherichia coli*. Explain why this drug is used for this type of infection. The following order has also been written for this patient: "Push fluids to 2000 mL/day." Explain the reason for pushing fluids.

CASE STUDY

Read the scenario and answer the following questions on a separate sheet of paper.

Virgil has been admitted to the medical unit and placed on aminoglycoside therapy as part of treatment for a urinary tract infection with *Pseudomonas*. He is 65 years old, awake, and alert, but anxious about his problem and wants to "hurry up and get better."

1. For which two serious toxicities will the nurse monitor, what are their symptoms, and how can they be prevented?

2. The physician adds penicillin to Virgil's drug regimen. Explain the reason for this.

3. Virgil's "trough" aminoglycoside level is 3.0 mcg/mL, and his serum creatinine level is increased from 2 days earlier. Are these results a concern? What should the nurse do? Explain.

Chapter 40

Antiviral Drugs

CHAPTER REVIEW

Choose the best answer for each of the following.

1. Acyclovir (Zovirax) is considered the drug of choice for treatment of infection with which of the following ?
   a. Cytomegalovirus (CMV)
   b. Human immunodeficiency virus (HIV)
   c. Respiratory syncytial virus (RSV)
   d. Varicella-zoster virus (VZV)

2. When administering ganciclovir HCl (Valcyte), the nurse keeps in mind that the main dose-limiting toxicity for this drug is which of the following?
   a. Kidney failure
   b. Gastrointestinal disturbance
   c. Peripheral neuropathy
   d. Bone marrow suppression

3. When reviewing the health history of a patient who is to receive foscarnet (Foscavir), the nurse knows that which condition would be a contraindication to its use?
   a. Renal toxicity
   b. CMV retinitis
   c. Asthma
   d. Immunosuppression

4. Amantadine would be used most appropriately in which of the following patients?
   a. A 29-year-old man who tests positive for HIV
   b. A 22-year-old woman who is in her eighth month of pregnancy and tests HIV positive
   c. A heart transplant patient who is to receive prophylaxis for influenza A
   d. An older adult patient who requires prophylaxis for influenza B

5. A patient calls the clinic nurse to ask for oseltamivir (Tamiflu) "because I was exposed to the flu over the weekend at a family reunion." The nurse knows that Tamiflu is indicated for which of the following? Select all that apply.
   a. Prevention of infection after exposure to influenza types A and B
   b. Reduction of the duration of influenza by several days in adults
   c. Treatment of topical herpes simplex virus infections
   d. Reduction of the severity of shingles symptoms

CRITICAL THINKING AND APPLICATION

Answer the following questions on a separate sheet of paper.

6. Why are so few antiviral drugs available? Why are viruses so difficult to kill?

7. Amy is 12 weeks into her pregnancy when she discovers that she is HIV positive. Amy is upset and says, "I won't live long enough to have this baby. We're both going to die." Is it possible to treat Amy and the fetus? Explain your answer.

8. Bailey, a 53-year-old teacher with osteoporosis, has shingles.

   a. What drug does the nurse expect the physician to prescribe?

   b. What instructions will the nurse give Bailey regarding any dietary considerations?

   c. Several months later, Bailey calls the office to say that her symptoms have returned. What action does the nurse expect to be taken now?

9. Brenda is a 5-year-old who has bronchopneumonia caused by RSV.

   a. What antiviral drug is used to treat RSV?

   b. Brenda's mother wonders whether the treatment will be completed before Brenda's birthday, which is 2 weeks away. What does the nurse tell her?

10. Eduardo, a 25-year-old translator, has AIDS. He was treated with zidovudine (AZT) for several months, but now the physician has switched him to didanosine (Videx EC) powder.

    a. What frequently is the reason that patients are switched from AZT to another anti-HIV drug?

    b. What instructions does the nurse give Eduardo regarding administration of the didanosine?

    c. Should Eduardo discontinue the antacid he has been taking? Explain your answer.

11. The nurse overhears a co-worker explaining to a student nurse the procedure for administering acyclovir (Zovirax) intravenously. After the acyclovir is diluted in sterile water, the co-worker says, "We'll administer this over at least an hour." Should the nurse intervene? Explain your answer.

12. Stacey has had symptoms of influenza for 4 days and feels miserable. She calls the nurse practitioner in the clinic to ask for "that medicine, Tamiflu, that is supposed to make the flu symptoms better." Should Stacey receive this medication at this time? Explain.

CASE STUDY

Read the scenario and answer the following questions on a separate sheet of paper.

Mr. Cuomo, a 30-year-old stockbroker, has been diagnosed with genital herpes simplex type 2 (HSV-2) infection. The physician has prescribed topical acyclovir (Zovirax).

1. What patient teaching does the nurse provide to Mr. Cuomo regarding administration of this drug?

2. Mr. Cuomo asks the nurse how long it will take for the acyclovir to cure his herpes. What is her reply?

3. What else should the nurse discuss with Mr. Cuomo, who is married?

4. HSV-2 virus is closely related to which other viruses?

Chapter 41

Antituberculosis Drugs

CHAPTER REVIEW

Choose the best answer for each of the following.

1. During isoniazid (Dom-Isoniazid) therapy, the nurse will closely monitor results of which laboratory tests?
   a. Liver enzyme levels
   b. Hematocrit and hemoglobin level
   c. Creatinine level
   d. Platelet count

2. The nurse should include which of the following information in the teaching plan for a patient who is taking isoniazid?
   a. Urine and saliva may be reddish-orange.
   b. Pyridoxine may be needed to prevent neurotoxicity.
   c. Injection sites should be rotated daily.
   d. The medications should be taken with an antacid to reduce gastric distress.

3. Patients who are in the initial period of treatment for tuberculosis need to be taught to do which of the following? Select all that apply.
   a. Wash their hands and cover the mouth when coughing or sneezing to reduce the spread of tuberculosis.
   b. Throw away dirty tissues with care.
   c. Be sure to get adequate rest, nutrition, and relaxation.
   d. Skip medication doses occasionally if gastric distress occurs.

4. A patient with newly diagnosed tuberculosis asks the nurse how long he will need to take "all this medicine." How long may drug therapy as treatment for active tuberculosis need to last?
   a. 6 months
   b. 12 months
   c. 24 months
   d. A lifetime

5. Why are multiple medications used in the drug regimen for tuberculosis?
   a. It reduces the possibility of the organism becoming drug-resistant.
   b. It ensures a cure of the disease.
   c. This regimen will reduce symptoms immediately.
   d. Patient adherence is better with multiple medications.

CRITICAL THINKING AND APPLICATION

Answer the following questions on a separate sheet of paper.

6. Diane, a 33-year-old proofreader, has been prescribed prophylactic isoniazid treatment.

   a. What laboratory studies should be performed before the start of therapy? Why?

   b. After Diane has taken the isoniazid for 2 months, the physician significantly reduces her dosage of the drug. Why might that be?

7. Ms. Innes is undergoing antituberculosis therapy that includes streptomycin.

   a. How is streptomycin administered?

   b. For what adverse effects will the nurse monitor?

   c. Ms. Innes takes an oral contraceptive. Is that a concern with Ms. Innes's streptomycin therapy? Explain your answer.

8. Why would an eye examination be performed before instituting antituberculosis therapy?

9. Mr. Fiore, a 42-year-old marketing executive, is on antituberculosis therapy. During his first follow-up visit, he is evasive when the nurse asks him about his adherence to his therapy regimen. He does tell her that he has been busy lately, entertaining various patients "at everything from cocktail parties to big sit-down dinners."

   a. What issues should the nurse discuss with Mr. Fiore?

   b. Several weeks later, Mr. Fiore returns for another follow-up visit. On examination, the nurse sees no apparent signs of tuberculosis. How can Mr. Fiore's therapeutic response be confirmed?

10. Frannie is a homeless 68-year-old woman who lives in a shelter some of the time. She was diagnosed at the community health clinic with tuberculosis, and antituberculosis therapy has been instituted.

    a. What patient education issues are of particular concern in Frannie's case?

    b. Frannie is staying at the shelter and seems to be handling her medication regimen well, but one day she comes by the clinic to tell the nurse that she is afraid the medication may be bad for her. "Whenever I go to the bathroom, everything is reddish-orange," she says. What does the nurse suspect is going on, and what does he tell Frannie?

CASE STUDY

Read the scenario and answer the following questions on a separate sheet of paper.

George, a 73-year-old retired plant foreman, has been diagnosed with tuberculosis. Nursing assessment reveals a history of gout and diabetes. He also has a history of heavy drinking.

1. What considerations will the physician keep in mind when deciding on a first-line drug for George?

2. George tells the nurse that he has been told that he has a "liver problem." His medical record mentions that he is a slow acetylator. How does this affect his therapy?

3. How will his history of "heavy drinking" affect his therapy?

4. The nurse instructs George about taking vitamin B_6 along with the isoniazid therapy. When he asks her why this is necessary, what does she tell him?

Chapter 42

Antifungal Drugs

CHAPTER REVIEW

Match each definition with its corresponding term.

1. _____ Single-celled fungi that reproduce by budding

2. _____ One of the major groups of antifungal drugs; includes amphotericin B (Abelcet) and nystatin (Dom-Nystatin)

3. _____ A large, diverse group of eukaryotic, thallus-forming microorganisms that require an external carbon source

4. _____ One of the major groups of antifungal drugs; includes ketoconazole (Nu-Ketocon), miconazole, and clotrimazole (Canesten)

5. _____ A term for yeast infection of the mouth

6. _____ One of the older antifungal drugs that acts by preventing susceptible fungi from reproducing

7. _____ The oldest antifungal drug

8. _____ An antifungal drug commonly used to treat candidal diaper rash

9. _____ An infection caused by fungi

10. _____ Multicellular fungi characterized by long, branching filaments called *hyphae*, which entwine to form a mycelium

a. Thrush

b. Moulds

c. griseofulvin (Grisovin)

d. Mycosis

e. Polyenes

f. Fungi

g. Imidazoles

h. amphotericin B (Abelcet)

i. nystatin (Dom-Nystatin)

j. Yeast

Choose the best answer for each of the following.

11. Which of the following drugs would be used to treat thrush in an infant?
    a. amphotericin B (Abelcet)
    b. fluconazole (Diflucan)
    c. nystatin (Dom-Nystatin)
    d. miconazole (Monistat)

12. During an infusion of amphotericin B, the nurse monitors for adverse effects, which may include which of the following? Select all that apply.
    a. Abdominal pain
    b. Fever
    c. Malaise
    d. Diarrhea
    e. Chills
    f. Rash

13. A patient calls the gynecological clinic because she has begun to menstruate while taking medication for a vaginal infection. She asks the nurse, "What should I do about taking this vaginal medicine right now?" Which of the following would be the nurse's best response?
    a. "You should stop the medication until menstrual flow has stopped."
    b. " Just take the medication at night only."
    c. " You should stop the medication for 3 days, then start it again."
    d. "It's okay to continue to take the medication."

14. Which medication is often used as a one-dose treatment for vaginal candidiasis?
    a. ketoconazole (Nu-Ketocon)
    b. fluconazole (Diflucan)
    c. griseofulvin (Grisovin)
    d. imidazole

15. Which is the drug of choice for treatment of many severe systemic fungal infections?
    a. amphotericin B (Ambinsome)
    b. fluconazole (Diflucan)
    c. griseofulvin (Grisovin)
    d. terbinafine (TMS-Terbinafine)

CRITICAL THINKING AND APPLICATION

Answer the following questions on a separate sheet of paper.

16. Why are there so few oral and parenteral drugs to treat mycotic infections?

17. Mr. Kim has been diagnosed with cryptococcal meningitis, and the physician has prescribed fluconazole (Diflucan).

    a. Why did the physician choose this drug rather than one of the other imidazoles?

    b. The results of Mr. Kim's cerebrospinal fluid culture eventually come back negative. When he hears the good news, he says, "Great! I'm tired of taking this medicine." What is the nurse's response?

18. The physician is planning intravenous amphotericin B therapy for James.

    a. What guidelines does the nurse follow in diluting the drug?

    b. What adverse effects does the nurse expect James to experience? Explain your answer.

    c. Should the nurse stop the infusion if those effects occur? Explain your answer.

19. Lewis has a severe fungal infection for which the physician has prescribed ketoconazole (Nu-Ketocom). During the nursing assessment, Lewis tells the nurse that he hopes the infection will clear up soon because he is going on a cruise ship in a week and he plans to "party every night!" What patient teaching issues should the nurse discuss with Lewis?

CASE STUDY

Read the scenario and answer the following questions on a separate sheet of paper.

Sally, a 68-year-old hospital volunteer, has been diagnosed with pneumonia with invasive aspergillosis. She has been treated for 2 weeks without much improvement, and the physician is considering starting voriconazole (Vfend) therapy. Sally is also receiving a medication for treatment of a cardiac dysrhythmia.

1. What is the reason for starting voriconazole therapy now rather than earlier?

2. What consideration may arise depending on the cardiac medication she is taking?

3. What should be monitored while she is taking voriconazole?

Chapter 43

Antimalarial, Antiprotozoal, and Anthelmintic Drugs

CHAPTER REVIEW

Choose the best answer for each of the following.

1. Before beginning antiprotozoal therapy, the nurse should assess the patient for which of the following contraindications?
   a. Underlying renal, cardiac, thyroid, or hepatic disease and pregnancy
   b. Porphyria and glucose-6-phosphate dehydrogenase (G6PD) deficiency
   c. Glaucoma, cataracts, anemia, and petechiae
   d. Constipation, gastritis, and lactose intolerance

2. The nurse should warn the patient taking quinine sulfate (Quinine-Odan) about which possible adverse effect?
   a. Constipation
   b. Irritation to the gastrointestinal mucosa
   c. A metallic taste in the mouth
   d. Severe halitosis

3. A patient is taking quinine therapy for a mild case of malaria. The physician has decided to add a sulfonamide or tetracycline drug along with the quinine. When the nurse gives the patient the prescription for this new medication, the patient is upset about having to take "another pill." What is the nurse's best explanation for the second drug?
   a. "The antibiotic treats bacterial infections that accompany malaria."
   b. "The antibiotic reduces the severe adverse effects of quinine."
   c. "The antibiotic will help the quinine to work more effectively against the malaria."
   d. "The antibiotic therapy is also needed to kill the parasite that causes malaria."

4. Which drug is used mainly for the management of *Pneumocystis jirovecii* (formerly *Pneumocystis carinii*) pneumonia? Select all that apply.
   a. metronidazole (Flagyl)
   b. pentamidine
   c. primaquine
   d. pyrantel (Combantrin)
   e. praziquantel (Biltricide)
   f. atovaquone (Mepron)

5. Which of the following statements is true regarding anthelmintic therapy?
   a. The medication can be stopped once symptoms disappear.
   b. Anthelmintics are more effective in their parenteral forms.
   c. Anthelmintics are broad in their actions and can be substituted easily if one medication is not well tolerated.
   d. The medication must be taken exactly as ordered for the length of time ordered.

6. Which patient is at the highest risk of dying from a protozoal infection?
   a. A teenager with no health problems
   b. A patient with diabetes mellitus
   c. A patient who has had a kidney transplant
   d. A patient with a history of myocardial infarction

CRITICAL THINKING AND APPLICATION

Answer the following questions on a separate sheet of paper.

7. Professor Henson has just returned from a research sabbatical in Africa where she did not adequately protect herself from mosquito exposure; thus, she has contracted malaria.

   a. What kind of parasite causes malaria?

   b. Which drug is recommended if the parasite is in the exoerythrocytic phase of development?

   c. Describe the the exoerythrocytic phase.

8. Professor Henson's physician would like to prescribe the drug you identified in your answer to question 7. The nurse should assess this patient for which kind of contraindications?

9. Professor Henson's husband, who accompanied her on her trip, has more recently begun to develop signs of malaria. He is given chloroquine, a 4-aminoquinoline derivative. However, unlike his wife, Mr. Henson sees no diminishing of his symptoms. His strain of malaria appears to be chloroquine-resistant. What alternative(s) can the nurse suggest for Mr. Henson?

10. The medical clinic in which the nurse works has a full waiting room this morning. Patient A is being seen for an intestinal disorder that he acquired after swimming in Lake Ontario. Patient B has AIDS and is showing early signs of pneumonia. Patient C is being treated and evaluated on a regular basis for a sexually transmitted infection. Here is the nurse's challenge: All three patients have something in common in terms of the causes of their disorders.

   a. Describe what the commonality could be.

   b. Based on that commonality, predict what disorder, of those discussed in this chapter, each patient might have. (*Hint: One patient has giardiasis.*)

   c. Select the drug the nurse thinks the physician is likely to prescribe for each patient.

CASE STUDY

Read the scenario and answer the following questions on a separate sheet of paper.

Sandra, age 15, has been diagnosed with intestinal roundworm infestation, specifically ascariasis, after a visit to another country. The nurse is preparing to medicate her with pyrantel (Combantrin).

1. How is this infestation diagnosed?

2. What are the contraindications to therapy with pyrantel?

3. The recommended dosage for pyrantel is 11 mg/kg, up to a maximum of 1 g, in a one-time dose. If Sandra weighs 57 kg, what dose should she receive?

4. What are the expected adverse effects of this medication?

Chapter 44

Antiseptic and Disinfectant Drugs

CRITICAL THINKING CROSSWORD

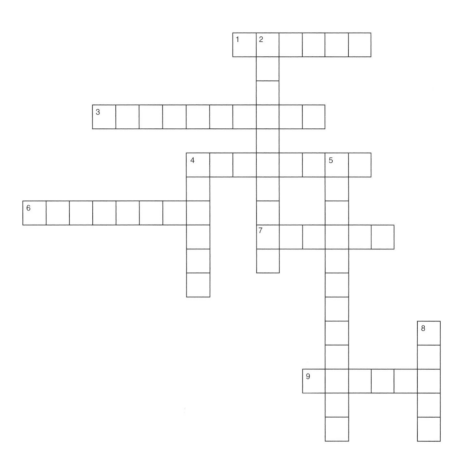

Across

1. Common trade name of benzalkonium chloride, a surface-active drug.
3. A type of infection also known as a "hospital-acquired" infection, acquired at least 72 hours after hospitalization.
4. The classification of glutaraldehyde.
6. One of the trade names of povidone-iodine, an iodine drug widely used as an antiseptic.
7. A nonmetallic element that readily forms salts with other elements.
9. One of the trade names of a sodium hypochlorite solution.

Down

2. A substance that inhibits the growth and reproduction of microorganisms without necessarily killing them.
4. An acid used in a 4–5% solution for killing microorganisms.
5. A chemical applied to nonliving objects to destroy microorganisms.
8. An example of a phenolic compound.

CHAPTER REVIEW

Choose the best answer for each of the following.

1. During a class on nosocomial infections, several facts are shared. Which of the following statements about nosocomial infections is true? Select all that apply.
   a. They are contracted in the home or community.
   b. They are contracted in a hospital or institution.
   c. They are more difficult to treat.
   d. The organisms that cause these infections are more virulent.

2. Which statement accurately describes the action of antiseptics?
   a. They are used to kill organisms on nonliving objects.
   b. They are used to kill organisms on living tissue.
   c. They are used to prevent the growth of organisms on nonliving objects.
   d. They are used to inhibit the growth of organisms on living tissue.

3. When preparing an area of skin before a procedure, the nurse knows that which strength of isopropanol (isopropyl alcohol) is most effective against microorganisms?
   a. 5%
   b. 25%
   c. 50%
   d. 70%

4. Before using povidone-iodine (Betadine) solution to prepare skin for surgery, the nurse should ask the patient about allergies to which of the following?
   a. Seafood
   b. Penicillin
   c. Mercury
   d. Milk

5. If a patient is allergic to povidone-iodine, the nurse may use which agent as a surgical scrub?
   a. Acetic acid
   b. Chlorhexidine gluconate (Hibiclens)
   c. Gentian violet
   d. Phenol

6. Which agent is used to disinfect surgical instruments?
   a. 5% acetic acid
   b. hydrogen peroxide
   c. glutaraldehyde (Cidex)
   d. Gentian violet

CASE STUDY

Read the scenario and answer the following questions on a separate sheet of paper.

A patient has been admitted to the hospital with an infected surgical wound in his groin area. The initial orders are for irrigation twice a day with hydrogen peroxide, then packing with gauze soaked with tincture of iodine. The hospital's wound care nurse reads this order, assesses the patient, then tells the nurse that she is going to call the physician for another order.

1. Why is the wound care nurse questioning this order?

2. The new order calls for irrigation with Dakin's solution, then wet-to-dry packing with saline. What is "Dakin's solution," and what concentration is appropriate for topical wound care?

3. The patient says, "That has a familiar smell. Why are you bleaching my wound?" What does the nurse tell him?

4. What should the nurse do after the dressing procedure is completed?

Chapter 45

Anti-Inflammatory, Antiarthritic, and Related Drugs

CHAPTER REVIEW

Choose the best answer for each of the following.

1. When teaching a patient about the common adverse effects of therapy with nonsteroidal anti-inflammatory drugs (NSAIDs), the nurse should mention which of the following?
   a. Dizziness
   b. Heartburn
   c. Palpitations
   d. Diarrhea

2. A 13-year-old has influenza, and her mother is concerned about her fever of 39.4°C. Which medication should the nurse suggest the mother use to treat the adolescent's fever?
   a. acetylsalicytic acid (Aspirin)
   b. acetaminophen (Tylenol)
   c. indomethacin (Apo-Indomethacin)
   d. naproxen (Anaprox)

3. A patient is receiving treatment with allopurinol (Alloprin) for an acute flare-up of gout. Which statements should be included in the patient teaching? Select all that apply.
   a. "Be sure to avoid alcohol and caffeine."
   b. "Take the medication with meals to prevent stomach problems."
   c. "You need to take this medication on an empty stomach to improve absorption."
   d. "You need to increase fluid intake to 3 L per day."

4. When reviewing the health history of a patient who is to receive NSAID therapy, the nurse should keep in mind that contraindications for the use of NSAIDs include which of the following?
   a. Pericarditis
   b. Osteoarthritis
   c. Bleeding disorders
   d. Juvenile rheumatoid arthritis

5. A patient receiving gold injections as treatment for arthritis should be told which of the following?
   a. Injections will be given via the intravenous route.
   b. The medication is more effective if fluids are restricted.
   c. Relief from symptoms can be expected in a few days.
   d. Relief from symptoms may take 3 to 4 months.

6. A young man is in the urgent care centre after experiencing a severe ankle sprain during a basketball game. The nurse expects that which pain reliever will be ordered for this patient?
   a. ketorolac (Torodol)
   b. acetylsalicytic acid (Aspirin)
   c. indomethacin (Nu-Indo)
   d. meloxicam (Dom-Meloxicam)

CRITICAL THINKING AND APPLICATION

Answer the following questions on a separate sheet of paper.

7. Ms. Jain is brought into the emergency room exhibiting the following symptoms: tinnitus, hearing loss, dimming vision, and dizziness. She is also thirsty and sweating profusely, and has had severe nausea and vomiting. On examination the nurse discovers that she has an increased heart rate and is experiencing some confusion. At first she appears drowsy, and then she begins to hyperventilate. The nurse suspects salicylism, but her colleague says, "No, this is acute salicylate intoxication." If he is correct, how was he able to tell? Differentiate between the cause of salicylism and acute salicylate intoxication.

8. Ms. Jain does have acute toxicity stemming from a salicylate overdose. Describe an appropriate treatment plan.

9. Mr. Chesney arrives at the emergency department with symptoms that are similar to Ms. Jain's but not as extensive. He is experiencing drowsiness, mental confusion, numbness, and disorientation, and had a seizure while en route to the hospital. What is wrong? What would the nurse expect if the situation was allowed to progress?

10. How will Mr. Chesney's treatment differ from Ms. Jain's?

11. Mr. Henry has come to the clinic complaining of a severe flare-up of his gout. He tells the nurse that he does not take his medicine on a regular basis because it "kills" his stomach. He also says he hates to take medicine yet hates the gout more. He has a prescription for allopurinol and a follow-up appointment for next week. What patient teaching would the nurse provide for Mr. Henry?

12. Eileen has had arthritic joint pain for months, and her current pain management has been less than successful. During a checkup today, she tells the nurse that she has heard of a new drug, Toradol, that "works wonders." She wants to try it for "a couple of months" to see if it can help her. What does the nurse tell her?

13. The nurse's neighbour calls him over to "check out this Aspirin bottle" that she found in her medicine cabinet. It has a strong vinegary odour. She wants to know if she can still take it for headaches. What does the nurse tell her?

CASE STUDY

Read the scenario and answer the following questions on a separate sheet of paper.

Sadie has been taking indomethacin as part of therapy for osteoarthritis but lately has noticed that it has been less effective. Her physician has decided to try celecoxib (Celebrex). Sadie has a history of hepatitis (15 years ago).

1. What advantages might there be to treatment with celecoxib rather than indomethacin?

2. What potential adverse effects should the nurse warn Sadie about before she takes this medication? What should she report?

3. Sadie asks the nurse if she can drink her usual glass of wine each evening while on this medication. What does the nurse tell her?

Chapter 46

Immunosuppressant Drugs

CHAPTER REVIEW

Choose the best answer for each of the following.

1. When monitoring patients on immunosuppressant therapy, the nurse must keep in mind that the major risk factor for patients taking immunosuppressants is which of the following?
   a. Severe hypotension with potential kidney failure
   b. Increased susceptibility to opportunistic infections
   c. Decreased platelet aggregation
   d. Increased bleeding tendencies

2. A patient is experiencing rejection of a transplanted organ. The nurse expects which drug to manage this?
   a. azathioprine (Imuran)
   b. cyclosporine (Neoral)
   c. muromonab-CD3
   d. tacrolimus (Advagraf)

3. A patient who is taking cyclosporine (Neoral) calls the office to say that he has heard that some food can increase the effectiveness of this drug. The nurse recognizes that he is talking about which of the following?
   a. Dairy products
   b. Orange juice
   c. Grapefruit juice
   d. Red wines

4. When teaching patients who are taking oral doses of immunosuppressants, the nurse should instruct the patient to do which of the following?
   a. Take them with food to minimize gastrointestinal upset.
   b. Take them on an empty stomach to increase absorption rates.
   c. Take them only when adverse effects are tolerable.
   d. Take them with antacids.

5. Patient teaching for those taking immunosuppressants should include which of the following? Select all that apply.
   a. The mouth and tongue should be inspected carefully for white patches.
   b. Allergic reactions to these drugs are rare.
   c. Patients should avoid crowds to minimize the risk of infection.
   d. Patients should report any fever, sore throat, chills, or joint pain.

6. Which of the following is the only immunosuppressant currently indicated for treatment of multiple sclerosis?
   a. glatiramer acetate (Copaxone)
   b. azathioprine (Imuran)
   c. basiliximab (Simulect)
   d. daclizumab (Zenapax)

CRITICAL THINKING AND APPLICATION

Answer the following questions on a separate sheet of paper.

7. Mrs. Flick is about to undergo heart transplant surgery. The physician plans to begin her on daclizumab (Zenapax).

   a. Mrs. Flick asks the nurse why. Explain how the nurse will answer her.

   b. Describe the laboratory studies to be performed and documented. How often should they be performed? What purpose do they serve?

   c. Three days before her surgery, an oral antifungal drug is added to Mrs. Flick's regimen. "Why do I have to take this, too?" Explain how the nurse will answer.

8. A patient on cyclosporine therapy is convinced that the cyclosporine is upsetting her stomach. What can be done to alleviate this problem?

9. Tess has had a kidney transplant. She is being given muromonab-CD3 intravenously, 5 mg/day in a single bolus. On the second day, she begins to exhibit chest pain, dyspnea, and wheezing. Her leukocyte count is 4×10^9/L. What is happening?

10. John has relapsing-remitting multiple sclerosis and is in the hospital because of an acute exacerbation. The physician talks to him about a "different type" of therapy with an immunosuppressant drug. What drug will be used, and how can it help John?

CASE STUDY

Read the scenario and answer the following questions on a separate sheet of paper.

Mr. Keller had kidney transplant surgery 6 months ago and so far has had no problems with organ rejection. He is taking cyclosporine (Neoral) in a maintenance dose. He wants to return to work and is in for a checkup before an approval is given for a return to his job.

1. He asks if he will have to continue the cyclosporine. What is the nurse's response?

2. He complains of difficulty swallowing, and as the nurse examine his mouth, she looks for signs of oral candidiasis. What findings would indicate that he has this condition?

3. After 2 weeks at work, Mr. Keller calls to report that he has influenza. He has a sore throat, chills, and aching joints, and he feels tired. What is the nurse's response?

4. When the nurse receives his most recent white blood cell count, she notes that the results are 2.9×10^9/L. Is this a concern, and what action, if any, will be taken?

Chapter 47

Immunizing Drugs and Pandemic Preparedness

CHAPTER REVIEW

1. **Complete the following chart by filling in all missing information.**

Drug	Active or Passive?	Purpose
a.	**b.**	Chicken pox
Hib	**c.**	**d.**
e.	Active	Hepatitis B virus prophylaxis
f.	**g.**	Postpartum antibody suppression
BCG vaccine	**h.**	**i.**
DTaP	**j.**	**k.**
Tetanus immune gloubin	**l.**	**m.**
Td	**n.**	**o.**

Choose the best answer for each of the following.

2. The immunity that is passed from a mother to her nursing infant through antibodies in breast milk is known as which type of immunity?
   a. Artificially acquired passive immunity
   b. Naturally acquired passive immunity
   c. Active immunity
   d. Immune globulins

3. Which of the following contain substances that trigger the formation of antibodies against specific pathogens?
   a. Antivenins
   b. Serums
   c. Toxoids
   d. Vaccines

4. When reviewing various immunizing drugs, the nurse recalls that some products provide long-lasting immunity against a particular pathogen. An example would be which of the following?
   a. Poliovirus vaccine, live oral
   b. Tetanus immune globulin
   c. Rh_0 (D) immune globulin
   d. Black widow spider antivenin

5. The nurse is preparing to give a second dose of DTaP vaccine to a 6-month-old infant. The infant's mother tells the nurse that the last time he recieved this vaccination, the injection site on his leg became warm, slightly swollen, and red. What is the nurse's best response?
   a. Explain that these effects can be expected, and give the medication.

b. Give one half the prescribed dose this week and the other half next week if tolerated well.

c. Skip the dose and notify the physician.

d. Wait 6 months, and then administer the dose.

6. A nurse has been stuck by a used needle while starting an intravenous line. Which preparation is used as prophylaxis against disease after exposure to blood and body fluids?

a. Hib vaccine

b. $Rh_0(D)$ immune globulin

c. Hepatitis B immune globulin

d. Hepatitis antitoxin

CRITICAL THINKING AND APPLICATION

Answer the following questions on a separate sheet of paper.

7. Jim, a cabinetmaker, is cut by a woodworking tool and comes to the clinic for stitches. When the nurse asks him about his tetanus vaccination history, he says, "I have no idea when my last tetanus shot was. I thought once I had all the shots for school that I was set for life! I don't need any more." What does the nurse explain to Jim?

8. Mrs. Krogg, an 82-year-old widow, is in the office for a follow-up appointment to evaluate her COPD. The physician recommends that she have an influenza virus vaccine. As the nurse prepares the injection, Mrs. Krogg says, "I had a flu shot last year. Why do I need another one this year?" What is the nurse's explanation to her?

9. Mr. Chao brings his toddler, Jordan, in for a 12-month well-child check. Before the nurse gives the measles-mumps-rubella (MMR) injection, what adverse effects does he tell Mr. Chao to watch for in Jordan's response to the immunization? What can be done to relieve these adverse effects?

10. Paul has received several immunizations in preparation for an overseas trip. He expected to feel some soreness at the injection sites, but the next morning he wakes up with swelling of the face and tongue, difficulty breathing, shortness of breath, nausea and vomiting, and a fever of 38.9° C. What is happening, and what should he do?

CASE STUDY

Read the scenario and answer the following questions on a separate sheet of paper.

The nurse is volunteering at a local animal shelter and helping to care for a sick dog that has just been admitted. During the examination, the dog nipped both him and the veterinarian. A while later, the veterinarian tells him that she fears that the dog has rabies and that both of them have been exposed. The veterinarian tells the nurse that she has had a vaccine for rabies but that he will need to be vaccinated immediately.

1. Is rabies a virus or a bacterium?

2. Did the vaccine the veterinarian received previously provide active or passive immunization? Explain.

3. Will the vaccine the nurse receives provide active or passive immunization? Explain why this particular type of vaccine is preferred in his situation.

4. How will the nurse's vaccine(s) be given?

Chapter 48

Antineoplastic Drugs Part 1: Cancer Overview and Cell Cycle–Specific Drugs

CRITICAL THINKING CROSSWORD

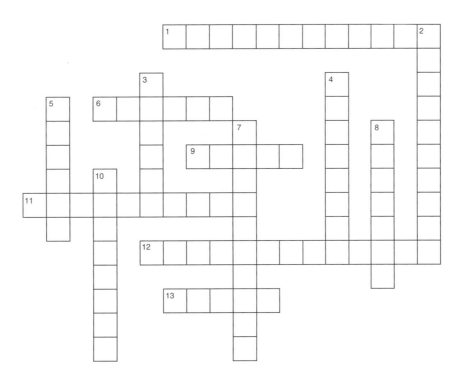

Across

1. During a pharmacology lecture, the instructor explains that some of the antineoplastic drugs have two reactive alkyl groups to alkalate two cancer cell DNA molecules. Thus, they are _____ drugs.

6. Mr. Kilpatrick's physician is not surprised to find that methotrexate is killing the cells of Mr. Kilpatrick's stomach, which results in nausea and vomiting. The methotrexate therapy is displaying a strong _____ potential in this patient.

Down

2. Mr. Kellogg has been treated with methotrexate for its folate-antagonistic properties. Now, however, he seems to be experiencing a toxicity reaction. The treatment he will receive will be _____ rescue.

3. Ms. Lilliankamp recently underwent a biopsy of a lump near her breast. Several days later, her physician calls and tells her that the lump is noncancerous and therefore is not an immediate threat to life. She is pleased to hear, then, that it is _____.

9. Mr. Schwartz is receiving methotrexate. The instructor asks for a full description of its mechanism of action, so you explain how it will inhibit dihydrofolic reductase from converting _____ acid to a reduced folate, thus ultimately prevent the synthesis of DNA and cell reproduction. The result, you explain, is that the cell will die.

11. Ms. Patchett had a biopsy performed on the same day as Ms. Lilliankamp (3 Down) did. When her biopsy specimen is analyzed, however, the results are the opposite of Ms. Lilliankamp's. That is, her lump is a(n) _____.

12. Mr. al-Filastini has just undergone a series of chemotherapeutic treatments when it is discovered that the antineoplastic drug has leaked into surrounding tissues; in other words, _____ of the drug has occurred.

13. Mr. Romano is interested in his chemotherapeutic process. As the nurse is discussing a drug's action, he hears the nurse use the term _____, and asks what it means. The nurse explains that this refers to the time frame at which the lowest neutrophil count occurs after administration of a chemotherapy drug that causes bone marrow suppression.

4. Ms. di Marco has a malignant neoplasm of the blood-forming tissues. Her bone marrow is being rapidly replaced with proliferating leukocyte precursors; she also has abnormal numbers (and forms) of immature white blood cells in her circulation, and even her lymph nodes, spleen, and liver are being infiltrated. Ms. di Marco's type of cancer is known as _____.

5. Mr. Harris is told that his cancer has metastasized. His physician explains to him that this means it has _____ to other areas of his body.

7. Mr. Blumstein has been diagnosed with chronic lymphocytic leukemia; Ms. Fehrers has multiple myeloma. Both patients will need treatment with a drug that can generate a reaction called _____, which, when it involves a cellular constituent such as DNA, will interfere with the cancer's mitosis and cell division of the cancer cells.

8. Mr. Pham is receiving an antineoplastic drug that has the ability to interfere with the process of cancer cell reproduction, which, if not halted, would result in the formation of two genetically identical daughter cancer cells containing the diploid number of chromosomes needed for its proliferation. In other words, the nurse explains, the drug will interfere with the cancer cells' _____ and cell division.

10. Ms. Fehrers has been given her first chemotherapy treatment. However, it soon becomes apparent that the adverse effects she is experiencing prevent her from being given dosages that will be high enough to be effective. These are dose-_____ adverse effects.

CHAPTER REVIEW

Choose the best answer for each of the following.

1. When administering antineoplastic drugs, the nurse needs to keep in mind that the general adverse effects of antineoplastic drugs include which of the following? Select all that apply.
   a. Bone marrow suppression
   b. Infertility
   c. Diarrhea
   d. Urinary retention
   e. Nausea and vomiting
   f. Stomatitis

2. A patient will be receiving chemotherapy with paclitaxel (Taxol). What should the nurse expect to do when administering this drug?
   a. Administer platelet infusions.
   b. Provide acetaminophen as needed.
   c. Keep the patient on "nothing-by-mouth" status.
   d. Premedicate with a steroid and antihistamines.

3. As the nurse is preparing to administer chemotherapy to a patient, the patient asks why more than one drug is needed. The nurse should explain that combinations of chemotherapeutic drugs are used to accomplish which of the following?
   a. Prevent drug resistance
   b. Reduce the incidence of adverse effects
   c. Decrease the cost of treatment
   d. Reduce treatment time

4. If extravasation of a neoplastic drug occurs, what should the nurse do first?
   a. Remove the intravenous catheter immediately.
   b. Stop the drug infusion without removing the intravenous catheter.
   c. Aspirate residual drug or blood from the tube if possible.
   d. Administer the appropriate antidote.

5. During chemotherapy, the nurse should monitor the patient for which of the following symptoms of stomatitis?
   a. Indigestion and heartburn
   b. Ulcerations of the mouth
   c. Severe vomiting and anorexia
   d. Diarrhea and perianal irritation

CASE STUDY

Read the scenario and answer the following questions on a separate sheet of paper.

Allen, a 40-year-old physician, has been diagnosed with acute lymphocytic anemia and will be receiving chemotherapy with methotrexate. He is scheduled to receive his first treatment today.

1. What is methotrexate's classification, and how does it work?

2. What laboratory test results should be checked before he receives this medication?

3. Allen tells the nurse that he often has problems with ankle pain from an old injury and takes ibuprofen (Motrin) for relief. Is this a concern?

4. What other medications may be given along with the methotrexate chemotherapy, and why?

Chapter 49

Antineoplastic Drugs Part 2: Cell Cycle–Nonspecific and Miscellaneous Drugs

CHAPTER REVIEW

Choose the best answer for each of the following.

1. While hanging a new infusion of a chemotherapy drug, the nurse accidentally spills a small amount of solution on the floor. The nurse's best action would be which of the following?
   a. Let it dry and then wipe up the floor.
   b. Wipe the area with a paper towel.
   c. Use a spill kit to clean the area.
   d. Ask the housekeeping staff to wipe the floor.

2. A patient is receiving leucovorin as part of the chemotherapy regimen. The nurse expects that the patient is receiving leucovorin to diminish the toxicity and counteract the effect of impaired _____ elimination.
   a. bleomycin (Blenoxane)
   b. cisplatin
   c. dactinomycin (Cosmegen)
   d. methotrexate

3. A patient receiving chemotherapy for a testicular tumour complains of hearing a "loud ringing sound" in his ears. The nurse expects that which of the following will happen next?
   a. The therapy will continue as ordered.
   b. The therapy will be stopped until the patient's hearing is evaluated.
   c. The therapy will be withheld for a day, and then resumed.
   d. The therapy will be stopped until renal studies are performed.

4. A patient is receiving outpatient chemotherapy. When teaching the patient about potential problems, the nurse needs to mention manifestations of an oncological emergency. Which of the following would the nurse include in his teaching? Select all that apply.
   a. Swollen tongue
   b. Alopecia
   c. Blood in the urine
   d. Nausea and vomiting
   e. Temperature of 37.8°C
   f. Chills

5. The nurse monitors closely for signs of liver toxicity when which neoplastic drug is given?
   a. doxorubicin (Myocet)
   b. cisplatin
   c. bevacizumab (Avastin)
   d. hydroxyurea (Hydrea)

6. A patient who has cancer is to receive a course of chemotherapy with doxorubicin. Which coexisting condition will require close monitoring while the patient is taking this drug?
   a. Hypertension
   b. Diabetes mellitus
   c. Gout
   d. Cardiomyopathy

CRITICAL THINKING AND APPLICATION

Answer the following questions on a separate sheet of paper.

7. Describe the concept of *cytoprotection* and provide some examples of how this may be accomplished during chemotherapy.

8. Mrs. Symthe has been receiving bleomycin to treat a lung tumour, and lately she has been experiencing increased difficulty breathing. She tells the nurse, "I guess this cancer is getting worse. The medicine is not working." Does the nurse agree, or is there another possible concern?

9. During a busy evening shift, a physician tells the nurse that he wants to start Mrs. Singh's chemotherapy immediately. The physician asks the nurse to mix the drug as soon as possible and start the infusion. Should she do this? Explain your answer.

10. Mr. Botolph, who has been receiving an infusion of mechlorethamine (Mustargen), has an infiltrated intravenous site. He wants the nurse to remove the intravenous line immediately because "it hurts so much." What will the nurse do? How will this extravasation be treated?

CASE STUDY

Read the scenario and answer the following questions on a separate sheet of paper.

Dottie, age 63, has been diagnosed with mid-stage ovarian cancer and will be receiving chemotherapy with cisplatin after surgery. She is anxious about the therapy but says that she wants to "beat the cancer."

1. Cisplatin is associated with three main toxicities. Describe each one.

2. Before Dottie receives the therapy, what should be assessed?

3. During therapy, Dottie complains of an "odd tingling" in her toes. Is this a concern? Explain.

4. Dottie tells the nurse that she would rather "drink nothing" when she is feeling nauseated. Is this a concern? Explain what the nurse needs to teach her about fluids.

Chapter 50
Biological Response–Modifying Drugs

CHAPTER REVIEW

Match each definition with its corresponding term. (Note: Not all terms will be used.)

1. _____ A type of cytokine that promotes resistance to viral infection in uninfected cells

2. _____ Cytokines that regulate the growth, differentiation, and function of bone marrow stem cells

3. _____ Cytokines that are produced by sensitized T lymphocytes upon contact with antigen particles

4. _____ An immunoglobulin that binds to antigens to form a special complex

5. _____ A substance that is foreign to the human body

6. _____ The primary functional cells of the cell-mediated immune system

7. _____ The specific cells of the humoral immune system

a. Colony-stimulating factors

b. Antibody

c. B lymphocytes (B cells)

d. T lymphocytes (T cells)

e. Interferons

f. Lymphokine-activated killer cells

g. Lymphokines

h. Antigen

i. Memory cells

Choose the best answer for each of the following.

8. When administering interferon drugs, the nurse knows that the best time to give them is at which of the following times?
   a. In the morning, before the patient rises
   b. At mealtimes
   c. Between meals
   d. At bedtime

9. A patient with a critically low hemoglobulin level and hematocrit is to receive a drug that will stimulate the production of red blood cells. The nurse expects that the patient will receive which of the following drugs?
   a. filgrastim (Neupogen)
   b. epoetin alfa (Epogen)
   c. pegfilgrastim (Neulasta)
   d. ferrous gluconate (iron)

10. While teaching a patient about the possible adverse effects of interferons, the nurse should include which of the following? Select all that apply.
    a. Myalgia
    b. Fever
    c. Diarrhea
    d. Fatigue
    e. Chills
    f. Dizziness

11. A patient is starting therapy with adalimumab (Humira) after a course of therapy with methotrexate failed to improve the patient's condition. The nurse recognizes that this patient is being treated for which of the following?
    a. Advanced-stage cancer
    b. Multiple sclerosis
    c. Severe rheumatoid arthritis
    d. Systemic lupus erythematosus

CRITICAL THINKING AND APPLICATION

Answer the following questions on a separate sheet of paper.

12. Dippy is to receive interferon as part of the treatment for cancer. Dippy is athletic and participates in sports activities on a regular basis. The physician explains that there is a dose-limiting adverse effect of this type of drug that may have a huge effect on her daily activities. What is this adverse effect, and how will it concern Dippy?

13. Konishi is receiving chemotherapy as part of his treatment for Hodgkin's disease. As she begins therapy, she tells the nurse, "I've seen those commercials about the drugs that increase your white blood cell count. Can't I start taking one of them now to keep my counts from getting so low?" What are the drugs that Konishi is referring to? How would the nurse respond to Konishi's question?

14. Michiko has received chemotherapy, and the results of today's laboratory work have indicated a critically low platelet count. He has received 2 units of platelets, but the physician has decided to give him a medication to improve his platelet counts. What drug will be given, and what concerns are there while his platelet count is so low?

CASE STUDY

Read the scenario and answer the following questions on a separate sheet of paper.

Connie, a 58-year-old woman, is in hospital for extreme weakness. She has received hemodialysis three times a week for chronic kidney failure for the last 2 years. The laboratory results revealed a critically low hemoglobin and hematocrit level, and the physician has ordered a transfusion of two units of packed red blood cells. However, Connie states that she cannot accept the blood transfusion because of her religious beliefs. As a result, there are orders to begin therapy with epoetin alfa (Epogen).

1. Explain the action of epoetin.

2. What laboratory test results should be monitored while she is taking this medication, and why?

3. Connie is concerned about the source of this drug. What can the nurse tell her about this?

4. Connie will be taking this drug at home. By what route will epoetin be given?

5. When Connie realizes that she will be giving herself injections up to three times a week, she complains, "Isn't there something else that I can take? I don't want that many shots!" Is there an alternative?

Chapter 51

Gene Therapy and Pharmacogenomics

CHAPTER REVIEW

Match each definition with its corresponding term. (Note: Not all terms will be used.)

1. _____ A structure in the nucleus that contains a linear thread of DNA that transmits genetic information

2. _____ A term for all of the chromosomal material within a cell

3. _____ The biological unit of heredity

4. _____ The complete set of genetic material of any organism

5. _____ The study of genomes, including the way genes and their products work in both health and disease

a. Allele

b. Gene

c. Genome

d. Genomics

e. Genetics

f. Chromatin

g. Chromosome

CRITICAL THINKING AND APPLICATION

Answer the following questions on a separate sheet of paper.

6. What is DNA, and what is its primary purpose?

7. What was the purpose of the Human Genome Project?

8. Name two effects of the Human Genome Project.

9. What is recombinant DNA, and how is this technology useful in pharmacology?

10. Explain the purpose of gene therapy. Has it been approved in Canada for routine treatment of disease?

Chapter 52

Acid-Controlling Drugs

CHAPTER REVIEW

Match each definition with its corresponding term. (Note: Not all terms will be used.)

1. _____ Drugs known as H_2 blockers that reduce stimulated acid secretion

2. _____ Drugs that block all acid secretion in the stomach

3. _____ A cytoprotective drug

4. _____ The cells responsible for producing and secreting hydrochloric acid in the stomach

5. _____ A type of antacid that can cause diarrhea

6. _____ Antacids that have constipating effects

7. _____ The cause of many peptic ulcers

8. _____ Drugs used to relieve the painful symptoms associated with gas

9. _____ A type of antacid that may contribute to the development of kidney stones

10. _____ A drug that can result in systemic alkalosis

a. Aluminum-containing antacids

b. Calcium-containing antacids

c. Magnesium-containing antacids

d. Antiflatulents

e. Proton pump inhibitors

f. *Helicobacter pylori*

g. Sodium bicarbonate

h. Histamine type 2 receptor antagonists

i. Sucralfate

j. Chief cells

k. Parietal cells

Choose the best answer for each of the following.

11. A patient with kidney failure wants to take an antacid for "sour stomach." The nurse needs to consider that some antacids may be dangerous when taken by patients with kidney failure, and should recommend which type of antacid?
    a. Activated charcoal
    b. Aluminum-containing antacids
    c. Calcium-containing antacids
    d. Magnesium-containing antacids

12. A patient with peptic ulcer disease will be starting medication therapy. He tells the nurse that he smokes and wonders if that will affect his treatment. The nurse's best response would be which of the following?
    a. "Smoking has no effect on these medications."
    b. "The actions of antacids are less potent when the patient smokes."
    c. "Smoking has been shown to decrease the effectiveness of H_2 blockers."
    d. "Smoking has been shown to increase the adverse effects of H_2 blockers."

13. Which drug class would be used as first-line therapy for gastroesophageal reflux disease that has not responded to customary medical treatment?
    a. H_2 blockers
    b. Antacids
    c. Mucosal protectors
    d. Proton pump inhibitors

14. Which of the following statements about proton pump inhibitors are true? Select all that apply.
    a. They should be taken 1 hour before antacids.
    b. They should be taken 30 to 60 minutes before meals.
    c. They should be taken with meals.
    d. They are part of the treatment of patients with *Helicobacter pylori* infections.
    e. There are few adverse effects with proton pump inhibitors.

CRITICAL THINKING AND APPLICATION

Answer the following questions on a separate sheet of paper.

15. The nurse's neighbour, Mr. Quang, comes over to get advice on antacids. He says he has taken Maalox "for years" for indigestion, but it is no longer working. He asks, "Can you recommend another antacid or one of those expensive, fancy pills that the pharmacy sells? Or should I just take baking soda?" What is the nurse's response?

16. Mrs. Knopf is advised to take omeprazole (Losec, Nexium) to treat her severe case of gastroesophageal reflux disease; nothing else has worked. Develop a patient teaching plan that will instruct Mrs. Knopf in how this medication should be taken.

17. Mr. McKinney has called to ask which antacid he should take. He has been to the store and is confused by the great variety on the shelves. He says he needs something for "occasional heartburn" when he eats something too spicy. He has a history of heart failure and is taking antihypertensive drugs. What type of antacid should he take, and what other instructions would he need?

18. Mr. Wolowski is taking enteric-coated aspirin for mild arthritis symptoms. He tells the nurse that he plans to take Aspirin with his favourite antacid, Maalox, because he does not want any stomach problems. What should the nurse tell him?

19. Frank has been diagnosed with a peptic ulcer caused by *Helicobacter pylori*. He has been told that he will be started on drug therapy for this disease. What does this involve?

CASE STUDY

Read the scenario and answer the following questions on a separate sheet of paper.

Eda, age 78, has been self-treating with antacids for "heartburn" for 6 months. After an upper gastrointestinal tract endoscopy, she was diagnosed with gastroesophageal reflux disease. The decision has been made to start treatment with cimetidine. Eda has been generally healthy except for a history of asthma. She says that she does not smoke but that she enjoys going to a bingo session every Saturday for a few hours where there is smoking, beer, and pizza.

1. When Eda sees the prescription for cimetidine, she asks, "Why do I need a prescription? I can buy this over the counter!" What does the nurse say in reply?

2. How will the cimetidine work to help gastroesophageal reflux disease?

3. What cautions, if any, are associated with the use of cimetidine?

4. Will staying in a smoke-filled room affect her therapy? Explain.

Chapter 53

Antidiarrheal Drugs and Laxatives

CRITICAL THINKING CROSSWORD

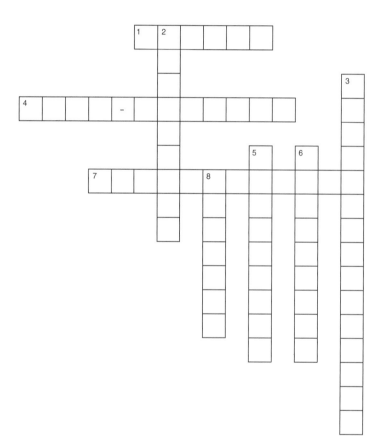

Across

1. Laxatives that increase osmotic pressure in the small intestine, increasing water content and resulting in distention.
4. Laxatives that absorb water into the intestine, increasing bulk and distending the bowel.
7. A laxative that increases fecal water content, resulting in distention, increased peristalsis, and evacuation.

Down

2. Acts by coating the walls of the gastrointestinal tract, binding to causative bacteria or toxin to allow elimination via the stool.
3. Acts by decreasing peristalsis and muscular tone of the intestine and thus slowing the movement of substances through the gastrointestinal tract.
5. Laxatives that softens the stool.
6. A laxative that stimulates the nerves that supply the intestine, which results in increased peristalsis.
8. Also act to decrease bowel motility.

CHAPTER REVIEW

Choose the best answer for each of the following.

1. Bismuth subsalicylate (Pepto-Bismol) would be the treatment of choice for which of the following patients?
   a. A 7-year-old child who has chickenpox
   b. A 23-year-old woman who has severe abdominal pain
   c. A 45-year-old man who is complaining of constipation
   d. A 58-year-old man who developed diarrhea after travelling outside of the country

2. Because of the possibility of toxicity, a patient who is self-treating with Pepto-Bismol should be told to avoid which of the following?
   a. acetylsalicytic acid
   b. acetaminophen
   c. calcium supplements
   d. vitamin tablets

3. A patient asks for a medication that will provide rapid relief of constipation. After ruling out possible contraindications, the nurse would suggest which of the following?
   a. psyllium fibre
   b. methylcellulose (Entrocel)
   c. docusate sodium (Colace)
   d. magnesium hydroxide (Milk of Magnesia)

4. A patient has been given PEG-3350 (Pegalax) as preparation for a colonoscopy. He began to have diarrhea after about 45 minutes. Two hours later, he tells the nurse that "the diarrhea has not stopped yet." What should the nurse do?
   a. Give him an antidiarrheal drug, such as diphenoxylate (Lomotil).
   b. Give him another dose of the PEG-3350 to finish cleansing his bowel.
   c. Remind him that it may take up to 4 hours to completely evacuate the bowel.
   d. Report this to the physician.

5. A 79-year-old patient visits the clinic today and tells the nurse that her "bowels just aren't right." She wants advice on the best laxative to take so that she can have a bowel movement every day. Which of the following are appropriate responses by the nurse?
   a. "A normal bowel pattern does not necessarily mean that you will have a bowel movement every day."
   b. "Try taking psyllium fibre with sips of water."
   c. "You can try taking Milk of Magnesia every day. It is considered a mild laxative."
   d. "Increasing fluids and fibre in your diet are better alternatives than laxative use."

CRITICAL THINKING AND APPLICATION

Answer the following questions on a separate sheet of paper.

6. Anna has called the health clinic in a panic. She says that she has been taking Pepto-Bismol for diarrhea and noticed this morning that her tongue "is a funny colour." She asks, "Have I overdosed on this stuff? What should I do?" What does the nurse tell Anna?

7. Mrs. Benedict is a 55-year-old store manager with osteoporosis and glaucoma. She has recently developed diarrhea, and the physician is considering antidiarrheal therapy. Mrs. Benedict tells the nurse that her husband recently "had a bout of diarrhea" for which he was prescribed a belladonna alkaloid. Mrs. Benedict wonders whether the same medication would help in her case. What does the nurse tell her?

8. Hillary has come to the physician's office complaining of constipation. During the nursing assessment, Hillary mentions that she recently started graduate school and has not had time lately to keep up her usual exercise regimen and that her diet is a "disaster." She says that on some days, all she has time to do is grab a milkshake at the student union. She also tells the nurse that she has been taking antacids for "heartburn." What might be causing Hillary's constipation?

9. Ira, a 45-year-old accountant, has chronic constipation.

   a. What are the advantages of bulk-forming laxatives in treating Ira's problem?

   b. The physician prescribes psyllium. What instructions does the nurse give Ira regarding its administration?

10. Drake is a 5-year-old boy with constipation. The physician has ordered treatment with glycerin suppositories.

    a. Why is glycerin a good choice for Drake?

    b. For what adverse effects will the nurse monitor?

11. Five-year-old Kyle has diarrhea, for which the physician has ordered an antidiarrheal drug.

    a. How will the dosage likely be determined?

    b. The next day, Kyle's mother calls to tell the nurse that Kyle seems to be no better and that his abdomen "looks bloated" and is painful. What is the nurse's action in this case?

CASE STUDY

Read the scenario and answer the following questions on a separate sheet of paper.

Charles, a 54-year-old accountant, recently completed a 2-week course of antibiotic therapy for pneumonia. He still has a slight cough but is now experiencing severe diarrhea.

1. What is the probable cause of his diarrhea?

2. What antidiarrheal drug is indicated for Charles?

3. How does this drug work?

4. Is this drug considered a drug or a dietary supplement? Explain.

Chapter 54

Antiemetic and Antinausea Drugs

CHAPTER REVIEW

Choose the best answer for each of the following.

1. Which drugs given to reduce nausea may cause drowsiness and drying of secretions?
   a. Antihistamines
   b. Neuroleptics
   c. Serotonin blockers
   d. Tetrahydrocannabinoids

2. Which class of antinausea drugs has proven to be effective in preventing chemotherapy-induced nausea and vomiting? Select all that apply.
   a. Antihistamines
   b. Neuroleptics
   c. Serotonin blockers
   d. Anticholinergics
   e. Tetrahydrocannabinoids

3. When reviewing the drugs used for nausea and vomiting, the nurse recalls that the drug which is a synthetic derivative of the major active substance in marijuana is which of the following?
   a. ondansetron (Zofran)
   b. metoclopramide HCl
   c. prochlorperazine (Nu-prochlor)
   d. dronabinol (Marinol)

4. A patient is undergoing chemotherapy. When giving antiemetics, the nurse will remember that these drugs are most effective against nausea when given at what time?
   a. Before meals
   b. At bedtime
   c. Before the chemotherapy begins
   d. Just after the chemotherapy begins

5. When giving dronabinol (Marinol) to a patient with AIDS, the nurse knows that this drug may also have what effect in addition to reducing nausea?
   a. Euphoria
   b. Enhanced appetite
   c. Reduced pain
   d. Enhanced sleep

CRITICAL THINKING AND APPLICATION

Answer the following questions on a separate sheet of paper.

6. Norman, who has Parkinson's disease, is experiencing nausea and vomiting. What class of antiemetic drug would *not* be a good choice for Norman, and why?

7. Petra has gastroesophageal reflux, and the physician has ordered oral metoclopramide.

   a. What instructions does the nurse give Petra for administration of the medication?

   b. A few days later, Petra calls to say that she thinks the medication is "too strong." She also mentions that her evening routine includes "a couple of glasses of wine." What does the nurse tell Petra?

8. Nellie, a patient on the nurse's unit, has been prescribed prochlorperazine (Nu-Prochlor) by intramuscular injection. She is on "nothing-by-mouth" status and has no intravenous access at this time. The nurse is preparing the injection when Nellie says, "I hate shots. Can't I just take it by mouth?" What alternatives are there for this drug, and what should the nurse do?

9. Chuck, a 33-year-old who is in a later stage of AIDS, has lost much weight and has no appetite. His doctor has prescribed dronabinol. When Chuck finds out that this medication is derived from marijuana, he becomes upset. "Why is the doctor giving me pot?" he asks. What does the nurse explain about this?

CASE STUDY

Read the scenario and answer the following questions on a separate sheet of paper.

Mr. Ontkin has been prescribed ondansetron (Zofran) during his chemotherapy, which is daily for 2 weeks.

1. For what significant drug interactions should the nurse assess before he takes ondansetron?

2. Mr. Ontkin tells the nurse that he still has nausea. He is puzzled because "I take the medicine for nausea as soon as I feel nauseated." What should she tell him?

3. One day, Mr. Ontkin complains to the nurse that he gets a headache every time the ondansetron is administered. What should she do?

Chapter 55

Pharmaconutrition

CRITICAL THINKING CROSSWORD

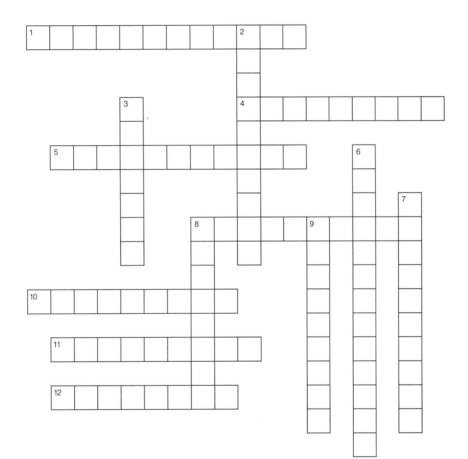

Across

1. Mr. Matabela is receiving _____ when it is determined that he is going to need nutritional supplementation as well. When the nurse sees that he is taking this drug, however, she asks if feeding can wait until his other drug therapy has run its course. She is concerned that the nutritional supplement will inactivate this drug because of high gastric acid content or prolonged emptying time.
4. Ms. Carter needs amino acids in nutritional supplements. The main use or primary role of amino acids is protein synthesis, or _____.

Down

2. When Ms. Carter asks why she needs amino acid supplemental feedings, the nurse explains that amino acids promote growth and help with wound healing. One of the principle ways they do so is by reducing or slowing the breakdown of proteins, or _____.
3. The Johnsons recently appeared in a television commercial because they drink Ensure to take care of a few extra nutritional needs they have experienced with aging. Their nephew recently had surgery; while recovering, he received nasogastric delivery of a modular formulation to supplement a polymeric feeding formulation

5. Mr. Ling is about to receive a _____, in which a feeding tube will be surgically inserted directly into his stomach.

8. Mrs. Vaschenko is worried about her husband, who has postsurgical nausea. She sees that his roommate is receiving total parenteral nutrition (TPN) and asks, "Can't you do that for my husband just while he's so nauseated?" TPN, the nurse explains, is to be used only when enteral support is impossible or when the gastrointestinal tract's _____ or functional capacity is insufficient.

10. Ms. Cedaras comes to the clinic when a cut on her hand "just won't heal up." She also says that as long as she is here, she would like to report symptoms of hair loss and scaly dermatitis. She wants a prescription for her skin problem, but the physician says, "There's something more going on here." He runs a few tests and discovers that Ms. Cedaras also has decreased platelets and some evidence of possible fatty liver. He says he suspects Ms. Cedaras has essential _____ deficiency (two words).

11. Mr. Manzini is having trouble getting and digesting enough dietary forms of amino acids. His physician explains that he needs nutritional supplementation through enteral nutrition to ensure that he gets enough of these amino acids, because they cannot be produced by his own body. Mr. Manzini is suffering from a deficiency of _____ amino acids.

12. Craig, a third-year university student, takes a great deal of interest in the supplementary nutritional product he is receiving and asks to read the label. He says, "There are some amino acids missing from this. Why aren't you giving me all of them?" The nurse explains that some amino acids (all but eight) are manufactured in the body, using _____ sources.

he needed. When their grandson was an infant, his parents supplemented his breastfeeding with an infant nutritional formulation. Each member of the Johnson family discussed here has received some form of _____ nutrition.

6. Lauren from 8 Down is receiving _____ amino acids.

7. The nurse is explaining to Mrs. Baranyai's family that the parenteral nutritional supplementation he is about to start will help her by bypassing the entire gastrointestinal system, eliminating the need for absorption, _____, and excretion.

8. Lauren, aged 10, is going through a period of rapid growth. She is receiving enough essential amino acids in her diet, and her body has no problems producing its normal levels of nonessential amino acids. Nevertheless, she is to receive two amino acids that are not produced in large enough quantities to support this rapid growth spurt. Lauren is to receive a supplemental source of histadine and _____.

9. Mr. Kennedy has been receiving peripheral parenteral nutrition. One day, something rather rare occurs: his vein becomes inflamed. The nurse notifies the physician. "Left untreated," she tells her, "this could have become really severe. He could even have lost his arm eventually if you hadn't caught this so quickly." Mr. Kennedy, of course, has _____.

CHAPTER REVIEW

Choose the best answer for each of the following.

1. The maximum concentration of dextrose in peripheral TPN infusions should be which of the following?
   a. 10%
   b. 20%
   c. 50%
   d. 100%

2. What are Ensure and Sustacal examples of?
   a. Elemental or monomeric solutions
   b. Blenderized solutions
   c. Polymeric, lactose-free solutions
   d. Polymeric, milk-based solutions

3. When monitoring a patient who is receiving TPN through a central line, the nurse should observe for complications, including which of the following? Select all that apply.
   a. Pneumothorax
   b. Aspiration
   c. Hyperglycemia
   d. Infection
   e. Air embolus

4. A patient who is just starting to take enteral nutritional supplements should be taught that the most common adverse effect the patient may experience is which of the following?
   a. Anorexia
   b. Constipation
   c. Diarrhea
   d. Flatulence

5. When reviewing a patient's need for nutritional supplementation, the nurse remembers that peripheral TPN is most appropriate for which of the following?
   a. Patients who will receive short-term TPN (for less than 2 weeks)
   b. Patients who will receive long-term delivery of TPN (for more than 2 weeks)
   c. Patients with severe nutritional problems
   d. Patients who wish to reduce their weight

6. Nursing interventions for patients receiving enteral feedings include which of the following?
   a. Checking gastric residual volumes once a day
   b. Starting the infusions at the maximum rate ordered
   c. Keeping the head of the bed flat
   d. Giving tube feeding formulas that are at room temperature

CRITICAL THINKING AND APPLICATION

Answer the following questions on a separate sheet of paper.

7. Ms. Schiller has one of the newer tubes being used for nasogastric feeding.
   a. What are the advantages and disadvantages of these newer tubes?
   b. What symptoms would she develop if she were lactose intolerant?
   c. Ms. Schiller's tube feeding rate is 50 mL/hr. After 24 hours, the nurse notes that the residual amount is 120 mL. What should the nurse do?

8. Mr. Robbins, who is on TPN therapy, has a weak pulse, hypertension, tachycardia, and decreased urine output. He seems somewhat confused, and the nurse notes, on examining him, that he exhibits pitting edema. What is wrong? Can the nurse do anything about it? What could the nurse have done differently to avoid this reaction?

CASE STUDY

Read the scenario and answer the following questions on a separate sheet of paper.

The nurse is caring for Mrs. Thomas, who is receiving peripheral parenteral nutrition via an intravenous (IV) line in her right forearm. The nurse's assessment shows that bag number 3 is infusing at 100 mL/hr via an infusion pump, and the bag has about 300 mL remaining. The site is intact, without redness or swelling.

1. Two hours later, Mrs. Thomas calls the nurse because she accidentally pulled the IV out of her arm. The remaining 300 mL of TPN has spilled on the floor. The nurse has tried to restart the IV but has not had success yet. What could occur if he cannot restart the infusion?

2. At last, the IV has been reinserted, but the nurse then discovers that bag number 4 has not yet been ordered from the pharmacy. What should he hang until bag number 4 is ready?

3. What else should the nurse monitor while Mrs. Thomas is receiving peripheral parenteral nutrition?

Chapter 56

Blood-Forming Drugs

CHAPTER REVIEW

Choose the best answer for each of the following.

1. Three days after beginning therapy with oral iron tablets, a patient calls the office. "I'm worried because my bowel movements are black!" What should the nurse do?
   a. Tell the patient to stop the iron tablets.
   b. Tell the patient to take the tablets every other day instead of daily.
   c. Ask the patient to come into the office for a checkup.
   d. Explain to the patient that this is an expected effect of the medication.

2. Patients who take iron preparations should be warned of the possible adverse effects, which may include which of the following?
   a. Dizziness and orthostatic hypotension
   b. Nausea, vomiting, diarrhea, and stomach cramps
   c. Drowsiness, lethargy, and fatigue
   d. Neuropathy and tingling in the extremities

3. What happens if folic acid is given to treat anemia without determining the underlying cause of the anemia?
   a. Erythropoiesis is inhibited.
   b. Excessive levels of folic acid may accumulate, causing toxicity.
   c. The symptoms of pernicious anemia may be masked, delaying treatment.
   d. Intestinal intrinsic factor is destroyed.

4. A patient is about to receive folic acid supplementation. The nurse knows that indications for folic acid supplementation include which of the following? Select all that apply.
   a. Megaloblastic anemia
   b. Tropical sprue
   c. Prophylaxis of fetal neural tube defects
   d. Pernicious anemia

5. When teaching the patient about oral iron preparations, the nurse will include which of the following instructions? Select all that apply.
   a. Mix the liquid iron preparations with antacids to reduce gastrointestinal distress.
   b. Take the iron with meals if gastrointestinal distress occurs.
   c. Liquid forms should be taken with a straw to avoid discolouration of tooth enamel.
   d. Oral forms should be taken with juice, not milk.

6. A patient asks the nurse, "What foods are good sources of iron? I know meat contains iron, but what other choices are there?" The nurse should suggest which of the following?
   a. Apples
   b. Citrus fruits
   c. Wheat crackers
   d. Raisins

CRITICAL THINKING AND APPLICATION

Answer the following questions on a separate sheet of paper.

7. Mr. Dlugy is prescribed intramuscular iron dextran. However, before the nurse can give him his first injection, the pharmacist suggests he give him a smaller dose of 25 mg first. Why does she suggest this? How should intramuscular iron dextran be administered?

8. The nurse is aware of the foods that contain iron. What other foods may either enhance the intake of iron or perhaps hinder it?

9. Four-year-old David has accidentally ingested an oral iron preparation, but he is not showing any adverse effects. Describe his treatment plan. If the serum iron concentration is higher than 54 micromoles/L, how is the treatment plan affected?

10. Describe the treatment of a child with more severe symptoms of iron intoxication than those seen in David (question 9). First describe the most severe intoxication symptoms of iron intoxication and then outline the treatment response.

CASE STUDY

Read the scenario and answer the following questions on a separate sheet of paper.

Maureen has been given ferrous fumarate capsules with instructions to take two capsules twice a day as part of her treatment for iron deficiency anemia.

1. She asks the nurse if she can take ferrous fumarate with meals. What is the nurse's answer?

2. What else should the nurse warn her to expect with this medication?

3. After a week, Maureen calls the nurse because she does not like to swallow capsules. She says that her mother has iron tablets that are labelled ferrous sulfate. She wants to know if she can take those tablets instead. What does the nurse tell her?

4. Because Maureen does not like the capsules, her iron preparation has been switched to an oral liquid suspension. While the nurse is teaching her how to give herself the correct dosage, what else is important to tell her about liquid iron preparations?

Chapter 57

Dermatological Drugs

CHAPTER REVIEW

Choose the best answer for each of the following.

1. Which of the following statements accurately describes antifungal therapy for topical infections?
   a. The length of treatment required to eradicate the organism may be from several weeks to as long as a year.
   b. Antifungal therapy works best when the affected area is exposed to sunlight.
   c. Oral drugs are the preferred drugs for treating topical fungal infections.
   d. Antifungal therapy is palliative only; fungi are rarely eradicated from topical areas.

2. When instructing a patient on how to use suppositories for vaginal yeast infections, the nurse should keep in mind which of the following?
   a. Suppositories should be inserted every other day at bedtime for 1 week.
   b. Suppositories should be inserted once daily at bedtime for 3 consecutive days.
   c. A one-time dose is administered in the morning.
   d. Suppositories should be inserted every night at bedtime until symptoms stop.

3. A patient has a painful sunburn that covers a large area of her body. To enhance the patient's comfort, the nurse can suggest that which of the following formulations be used for this patient's topical medication?
   a. Aerosol spray
   b. Gel
   c. Oil
   d. Cream

4. Ms. Thierry needs a medication that has excellent emollient properties. Because she works as a swimming coach, the medication prescribed should not wash off when it comes in contact with water. If each has the same healing properties, which of the following formulations would be preferred for Ms. Thierry?
   a. Aerosol spray
   b. Gel
   c. Oil
   d. Cream

5. Which of the following statements about topical antiviral drugs are true? Select all that apply.
   a. Common adverse effects include stinging, itching, and rash.
   b. Topically applied acyclovir does not cure viral skin infections but does seem to decrease the healing time and pain.
   c. Topically applied acyclovir (Zovirax) can cure viral skin infections if applied as soon as symptoms appear.
   d. Antiviral drugs are applied topically for the treatment of both initial and recurrent herpes simplex infections.

6. Beatrix, age 22, is taking isotretinoin (Accutane) as part of the treatment for severe cystic acne. Which of the following is part of the patient teaching she will require?
   a. Isotretinoin reduces acne by causing skin peeling.
   b. Isotretinoin's use is contraindicated if she is allergic to erythromycin.
   c. Beatrix will need to apply it twice a day to her face, after washing her face thoroughly.
   d. Beatrix will need to use two forms of birth control while taking this medication.

CRITICAL THINKING AND APPLICATION

Answer the following questions on a separate sheet of paper.

7. Mr. Mugler has a topical skin infection. He is prescribed clindamycin. He has never used this drug before. The nurse realizes that it is a good idea to assess him for possible sensitivity or allergies. What precautions can the nurse take?

8. The nurse is getting ready to apply erythromycin to a patient's skin. The affected area of the skin is not oozing or even moist, but her supervisor still requires that she wear gloves. Why?

9. Mr. Lacroix's two children have brought "something" home from school, and within a day, he had "it," too. He tells the nurse he has applied lindane (Hexit) to everyone's scalps, but he has come to the clinic to have his children and himself checked because he is not confident that he has "taken care of things properly." What are Mr. Lacroix and his children being treated for? Describe for him the basic steps in using lindane. What other measures should he take?

10. With a partner, develop two different case studies of acne patients. Assign one patient to take benzoyl peroxide (Acetoxyl) and the other tretinoin (Retin-A). What differences in implementation and precautions do you come up with for the two patients?

CASE STUDY

Read the scenario and answer the following questions on a separate sheet of paper.

Judy is in the clinic today because she burned her arm last evening while frying chicken. She has a second-degree burn over a 12.7 cm area of her forearm. She did not apply anything to it overnight, and the wound is reddened and peeling.

1. The physician tells the nurse that he is going to apply silver sulfadiazine cream to the site. What will he need to do before applying this cream?

2. He tells Judy that the area will need to be kept covered. Why is this necessary?

3. As the physician prepares to apply the cream, the nurse notices that he is about to reach into the medication jar with his ungloved fingers. Is this okay?

4. Are there any adverse effects associated with this medication?

Chapter 58

Ophthalmic Drugs

CHAPTER REVIEW

Match each definition with its corresponding term. (Note: Not all terms will be used.)

1. _____ Adjustment of the lens to variation in distance

2. _____ Inflammation of the eyelids

3. _____ The clear, watery fluid that circulates in the anterior and posterior chambers of the eye

4. _____ An abnormal condition of the lens of the eye, characterized by loss of transparency

5. _____ Paralysis of the ciliary muscles, which prevents accommodation of the lens to variations in distance

6. _____ Excessive intraocular pressure caused by elevated levels of aqueous humor

7. _____ The mucous membrane that lines the eyelids

8. _____ Drugs that constrict the pupil

9. _____ The vascular middle layer of the eye, containing the iris, ciliary body, and the choroid

10. _____ Drugs that dilate the pupil

a. Cycloplegia

b. Conjunctiva

c. Accommodation

d. Glaucoma

e. Mydriatics

f. Miotics

g. Uvea

h. Blepharitis

i. Vitreous humor

j. Aqueous humor

k. Cataract

Choose the best answer for each of the following.

11. When reviewing the medical record of a patient with a new order for a carbonic anhydrase inhibitor, the nurse knows that which condition would be a potential problem for a patient taking this drug?
    a. Glaucoma
    b. Ocular hypertension
    c. Allergy to sulfa drugs
    d. Allergy to penicillin

12. During an ophthalmic procedure, the patient receives ophthalmic acetylcholine. The nurse is aware that the purpose of this drug is which of the following?
    a. To produce mydriasis for ophthalmic examinations
    b. To produce immediate miosis during ophthalmic surgery
    c. To cause cycloplegia to allow for measurement of intraocular pressure
    d. To provide topical anaesthetic during ophthalmic surgery

13. When administering latanoprost (Xalatan) eye drops, the nurse should advise the patient of which of the following possible adverse effects?
    a. Temporary eye colour changes, from light eye colours to brown
    b. Permanent eye colour changes, from light eye colours to brown
    c. Photosensitivity
    d. Bradycardia and hypotension

14. Willis has come to the emergency room with an eye injury. After the application of fluorescein, the physician sees an area with a green halo. What does this indicate?
    a. A corneal defect
    b. A conjunctival lesion
    c. The presence of a hard contact lens
    d. A foreign object

15. When applying ophthalmic drugs, the nurse should follow which instructions? Select all that apply.
    a. Apply drops directly onto the cornea.
    b. Apply drops into the conjunctival sac.
    c. Apply pressure to the inner canthus for 1 minute after medication administration.
    d. Apply ointments in a thin layer.

16. To prevent gonorrheal eye infection, a newborn infant will receive which of the following?
    a. dexamethasone (Maxidex) ointment
    b. gentamicin (Diogent) ointment
    c. erythromycin (AK Mycin) ointment
    d. sulfacetamide/prednisolone (AK Cide) solution

CRITICAL THINKING AND APPLICATION

Answer the following questions on a separate sheet of paper.

17. Jonathan has blue eyes; Julie has brown eyes. Why would the drug effects of miotics on the iris be less pronounced in Julie?

18. Mrs. Ngo, 60 years old, has open-angle glaucoma. The physician prescribes dipivefrin (Propine).

    a. Why might this drug be chosen over epinephrine (Epifrin) ?

    b. What problems does the nurse expect Mrs. Ngo to report?

    c. Does the nurse expect any serious reactions to the drug? Explain your answer.

19. The physician prescribes a β-adrenergic blocker for Ned, who has ocular hypertension. Ned experiences what he calls "an allergic reaction" to the drug. Consequently, the physician changes Ned's medication to another β-blocking drug, timolol (Tim-AK). Because both of these drugs are β-adrenergic blockers and Ned had a reaction to the first drug, why would the physician simply switch Ned to another drug in the same category?

20. Mrs. O'Rourke, who has open-angle glaucoma, has been scheduled for laser surgery.

    a. What drugs could be used?

    b. What is an adverse effect of these drugs?

21. Louisa has an inflammatory disorder of the eye, for which the physician has prescribed a topical nonsteroidal anti-inflammatory ophthalmic drug. Why might the physician have chosen an NSAID over a corticosteroid?

22. Ms. Luna has been prescribed ophthalmic corticosteroid drops for an inflammation of her eye. The next day, she calls the clinic and tells the nurse, "These drops sting so much when I use them that I can't even put in my contacts." What would the nurse explain to Ms. Luna?

CASE STUDY

Read the scenario and answer the following questions on a separate sheet of paper.

Mr. Djukic has developed a viral ocular infection, cytomegalovirus (CMV) retinitis, after being diagnosed with AIDS 6 months ago.

1. He is upset about his eye infection. He says he has been meticulous with his health and hygiene since his diagnosis and does not understand how he got this ophthalmic infection. What can the nurse tell him?

2. What method of medication delivery is used to treat this infection?

3. The opthalmologist decides to use ganciclovir HCl (Valcyte) to treat Mr. Djukic's infection. How will this drug be started?

4. Mr. Djukic asks the nurse how long this medication will be needed. What does the nurse tell him?

Chapter 59

Otic Drugs

CHAPTER REVIEW

Choose the best answer for each of the following.

1. When assessing for otitis media, the nurse recalls that common symptoms of this condition include which of the following? Select all that apply.
   a. Pain
   b. Malaise
   c. Ear drainage
   d. Hearing loss
   e. Fever

2. A patient with a middle ear infection will generally require treatment with which of the following?
   a. Topical steroids
   b. Systemic steroids
   c. Topical antibiotics
   d. Systemic antibiotics

3. An elderly patient has a buildup of cerumen in his left ear. The nurse expects that this patient will receive which type of drug for this problem?
   a. Antifungal
   b. Wax emulsifier
   c. Steroid
   d. Local analgesic

4. Before giving ear drops, the nurse checks for contraindications to the use of otic preparations, such as which of the following?
   a. Eardrum perforation
   b. Infection
   c. The presence of cerumen
   d. Mastoiditis

5. In children, what usually precedes episodes of otitis media?
   a. Participation in a swim team
   b. Injury from a foreign object
   c. Upper respiratory tract infection
   d. Mastoiditis

CRITICAL THINKING AND APPLICATION

Answer the following questions on a separate sheet of paper.

6. A patient calls the physician's office complaining of severe pain in and drainage from his left ear. He also says he "had a little mishap" on his motorcycle yesterday. What does the nurse tell him?

7. Why are anti-infective drugs frequently combined with steroids?

8. André, a 30-year-old teacher, has an ear infection and a prescription for ear drops.

   a. What does the nurse do before she instill the drops?

   b. What does the nurse warn André might happen after the drops are instilled?

9. Mrs. Franz, a 52-year-old office manager, has come to the clinic today complaining of a painful, "itchy" left ear. The physician diagnoses an infection of the external auditory canal and prescribes a topical antibiotic.

   a. What is the advantage of using a product containing hydrocortisone?

   b. What would be a contraindication to Mrs. Franz's use of this type of drug?

10. Why do so many otic combination products contain local anaesthetic drugs?

11. Ben is a 2-year-old who attends day care, and his brother Drew is a 6-year-old in kindergarten. They both require otic drugs for ear infections.

    a. What instructions does the nurse give the boys' parents regarding instillation of the drops?

    b. A few days after they are first seen, the boys' mother brings them back for a follow-up visit. Ben and Drew do not seem to be in pain, and there is no redness or swelling in either child's ears. What does this mean?

12. During a home visit, the nurse observe Esther's husband preparing her ear drops. He puts a glass of water in the microwave, telling the nurse that he will soak the bottle of ear drops in hot water to warm them up.

    a. How is Esther's husband doing so far?

    b. Later, immediately after her husband instills the drops, Esther sits up and asks the nurse whether they are now doing everything right. What does the nurse tell her?

CASE STUDY

Read the scenario and answer the following questions on a separate sheet of paper.

Mark, who is 45 years old, is in the office complaining of a "heavy" feeling in his left ear, along with slight pain and decreased hearing. When the nurse walks into the examination room, she finds Mark inserting a cotton-tipped applicator into his ear "to scratch it."

1. What does the nurse suspect is the problem with his ears?

2. What can be done to address this problem?

3. The nurse gives Mark a container of urea hydrogen peroxide (Murine Ear Drops). Before she continues, he asks her how many times a day he needs to take this medication and whether he can take it with meals. How is this medication given?

4. Other than Murine Ear Drops, what is (are) the alternative(s) to loosen wax buildup in the ear?

Overview of Dosage Calculations

Disclaimer: *Please note that the drugs and dosages within this chapter are examples, for educational purposes only; please refer to appropriate drug resources for dosage information.*

Accurate drug calculation skills are important, as a mistake in calculating can result in a medication error that causes unwanted consequences for the patient. There are many important aspects to consider when doing calculations, but the most important one may be common sense. If a drug dose calculation does not seem right, then most likely it is not. The administration of drugs to patients is a shared responsibility among the patient, physician, pharmacist, and nurse. All those involved have moral, ethical, and legal responsibilities to ensure that the administration of drugs takes place in a safe and effective way. The nurse has both a legal and a professional responsibility to ensure that his or her patients receive the right dose of the right drug at the right time and by the right route. There are many checks and balances in the system to guarantee that this happens. The necessary basic calculations involved in the safe and accurate administration of medications to patients are described in this section.

Calculating drug doses is one part of the overall process of pharmacological therapy. Before actually calculating a drug dose, the nurse must follow several steps. The nurse should assess the patient and the prescribed medication according to the traditional "5 rights": right patient, right drug, right dose, right time, and right route. Other principles to follow to decrease the likelihood of mistakes are to calculate doses systematically and to do the calculations consistently time after time so that the process becomes easier with each calculation. It also helps to have a peer check the calculations, especially if the dose seems unusual or the math is difficult. Remember, common sense should prevail. If a calculation shows that you should give 25 mg of digoxin and the strongest strength is 0.25 mg, common sense should tell you that the patient should not be given 100 pills, especially since drug dosage forms are usually manufactured with the most commonly prescribed dosages in mind.

You must have basic arithmetic skills before beginning. The following basic principles may need to be reviewed:

➢ Basic multiplication
➢ Basic division
➢ Roman numerals
➢ Fractions (reducing to lowest terms, addition, subtraction, multiplication, division, mixed numbers)
➢ Decimals (adding, subtracting, multiplication, division)
➢ Ratios and percentages (changing a fraction to a percentage, changing a ratio to a percentage)
➢ Solving for "x" in a simple equation

RULES TO REMEMBER

❖ Before calculating a drug dose for a particular patient, you must first convert all units of measure to a SINGLE system, if this has not already been done. The best approach is to convert to the system used on the drug label. Although metric is the preferred system in Canada, it may still be necessary to convert the patient's weight from pounds to kilograms if the medication is ordered to be given per kilogram of weight.

Rounding

❖ Always round your answers to the nearest dose that is *measurable*, after verifying that the dose is correct for that patient.
  • If a tablet is scored, you may round to the nearest half tablet.
    Example: 1.8 tablets, give 2 tablets
    1.2 tablets, give 1 tablet
  • If a tablet is unscored, call the pharmacy to check if there is a lower dosage tablet available, or if a pill cutter is suitable to use to split the pill. It is difficult to cut an unscored tablet into fourths accurately. Remember that enteric-coated, sustained-release, or extended-release formulations cannot be cut or crushed!
  • Recheck your calculations if the dose is more than one or two tablets.
  • To round liquids, *look at the equipment you plan to use*. Some syringes are marked in tenths or hundredths of a millilitre. Larger syringes are marked in 0.2-mL increments. Tuberculin syringes are marked in one-hundredths. For liquid medications, NEVER round up to the nearest WHOLE number. If the

answer is 1.8 mL, DO NOT round up to 2 mL. Rounding up in these situations may lead to overdosing. However, if you are using an electronic infusion pump, you will probably need to round to the nearest whole number.

- To round to the nearest tenth, look at the hundredths column. If it is 0.5 or more, round UP to the next tenth.
  Example: To round to the nearest tenth:
  1.78 or 1.75, round to 1.8
  1.32 or 1.34, round to 1.3
- A syringe calibrated in hundredths permits more exact measurement of small dosages. To round to the nearest hundredth, look at the thousandth column. If it is 0.005 or more, round UP to the next hundredth.
  Example: To round to the nearest hundredth:
  1.847, round to 1.85
  1.653, round to 1.65
- **NOTE:** Never round up liquid medications to the nearest whole number. If the answer is 1.6 mL, DO NOT round up to 2 mL! Such increases may lead to overdoses.
- **CHILDREN'S DOSES** are rounded to the **TENTHS** place, not whole numbers. Rounding to whole numbers may lead to overdoses.

Leading Zeros

❖ Always insert a zero (0) in front of decimals when the number is less than a whole number. This draws attention to the decimal and avoids potential errors.

Example: 0.05 is CORRECT
.05 is NOT correct

Trailing Zeroes

❖ Never place a lone zero after a decimal point. If the decimal is not noticed, a dangerous dosage error may occur.
Example: 3 is CORRECT
3.0 is NOT correct and may be mistaken for 30

Labelling

❖ Always label your answers with the appropriate unit. If the problems asked for a number of tablets, write "tablets." If you are to give an injection, use "mL." For heparin and insulin, however, use "units" instead of "mg" or "mcg." Intravenous drips will be written in terms of "mL/hour." Problems using an intravenous infusion pump are ALWAYS asking for mL/hr. THINK about what the question is asking, and then label your answer appropriately.

Common Sense

❖ Use common sense! Drug companies typically formulate medications that are close to the usual doses and medications that can provide the ordered dose with one or two tablets. If your answer indicates that you should give 60 mL intramuscularly, CHECK IT AGAIN! Remember, you can only give 2 to 3 mL intramuscularly, depending on institution policies, so a dosage of 60 mL would be inappropriate.

INTERPRETING MEDICATION LABELS

Medication labels contain a tremendous amount of information, much of it in small print. The drug manufacturer prints some labels; others are prepared by pharmacy technicians or pharmacists for institutional use. The most important information is as follows:

- Generic name—the first letter is lower-cased. This is the name used by all companies that produce the drug.
- Trade, brand, or proprietary name—the first letter is usually capitalized. This name is used only by the manufacturer of the drug and may be followed by the "®" symbol.
- Drug Identification Number (DIN)—a "computer-generated eight digit number assigned by Health Canada to a drug product prior to being marketed in Canada. It uniquely identifies all drug products sold in a dosage form in Canada and is located on the label of prescription and over-the-counter drug products that have been evaluated and authorized for sale in Canada" (Health Canada, 2009).
- Unit dose per millilitre, per tablet, per capsule, and so on
- Total amount in the container

- Route
- Directions for preparation, if needed
- Directions for storage
- Expiration date

Other information, such as a specification for adult or child use, may be noted on the label.

Example:

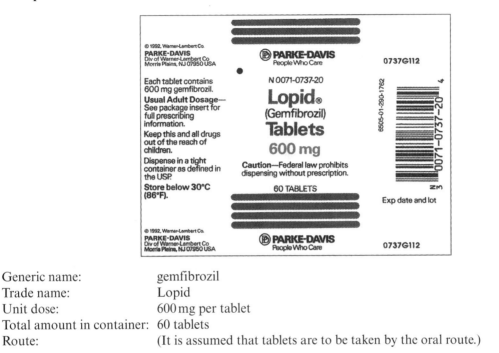

Generic name:	gemfibrozil
Trade name:	Lopid
Unit dose:	600 mg per tablet
Total amount in container:	60 tablets
Route:	(It is assumed that tablets are to be taken by the oral route.)

For the following labels, identify the information requested.

1.

Generic name: _____
Trade name: _____
Unit dose: _____
Total amount in container: _____
Route: _____

2.

Generic name: _____
Trade name: _____
Unit dose: _____
Total amount in container: _____
Route: _____

SECTION I: BASIC CONVERSIONS USING RATIO AND PROPORTION

A proportion is a way of stating a relationship of equality between two ratios. The first ratio listed is EQUAL to the second ratio listed. The double colon (::) that separates the two ratios means AS. The numbers at each end of the ratio equation can be called the "outside," and the two numbers in the middle of the ratio (around the "::") can be called the "inside." Ratio and proportion problems can be used to calculate ONE of the numbers in the equation if it is not known. The simple rule to use is this:

The product of the outside terms equals the product of the inside terms.

If one of the terms is not known, it is designated as "x." The problem is then set up to solve for "x."

Example:

1 : 100 :: 4 : x means:
"The relationship of 1 to 100 is the same as the relationship of 4 to x." The "x" is unknown.

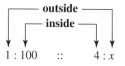

1 and x are the "outsides;" 100 and 4 are the "insides." To solve for x, multiply the outsides (1 × x) together, multiply the insides (100 × 4) together, and form an equation:

(1 × x) = (100 × 4)
$1x$ = 400
x = 400

Proof: You may prove your equation as follows: Insert the answer for x in the original equation, then solve.

1 × 400 = 400 (outsides)
100 × 4 = 400 (insides)
400 = 400; the answer for x is correct.

Example:

5 : 25 :: 15 : x
Multiply the outsides and the insides and form an equation; then solve for x.
(5 × x) = (25 × 15)
$5x$ = 375
x = 375/5
x = 75

Proof:

5 × 75 = 375
25 × 15 = 375
375 = 375

Calculating ratios is one of the major foundations of drug dosage calculations. When calculating a dosage, the nurse will use the medication on hand to calculate how much of it to give for a desired dosage. The nurse uses the principle of proportion to calculate accurately how much medication to give. The following chart provides a few common equivalents used in pharmacology. These equivalents are then used in ratio and proportion problems to calculate appropriate dosages.

BASIC EQUIVALENTS

Metric Equivalent	Approximate Equivalent
Weight 1 mg = 100 µg or mcg (micrograms) 1 g = 1000 mg (milligrams) 1 kg = 1000 g (grams) **Volume** 1000 mL = 1 L	1 tsp = 5 mL 1 tbsp = 15 mL 2 tbsp = 30 mL 1 oz = 30 mL 1 kg = 2.2 lb 1 mL (weighs approximately 1 g)

To find basic equivalents from one unit of measure to another, use the ratio and proportion approach.

Example 1: The drug dosage is 500 mg. You have scored tablets on hand that are 1 g each. How many tablets will you give?

You have *grams* on hand. You need to change the *milligrams* needed to the equivalent *grams* on hand. Find the proper equivalents:
Equivalent: 1 g = 1000 mg
Next, set up the ratio and proportion equation.
On the LEFT side put the ratio that you **know:** 1 g is 1000 mg
On the RIGHT side, put the ratio that you **want to know:** how many g ("x") is 500 mg?

Know   **Want to Know**
1 g : 1000 mg :: x g : 500 mg
Solve for x: $(1 \times 500) = (1000 \times x)$; $500 = 1000x$; $x = 500/1000$; $x = 0.5$
You will give 0.5 (half) of the 1 g tablet.
To double-check your answer, substitute your answer for the x and solve. The outsides should equal the insides.
$1 \times 500 = 500$; $1000 \times 0.5 = 500$; $500 = 500$

Example 2: Mabel weighs 122 lb. How many kilograms does she weigh?

Equivalent: 1 kg = 2.2 lb

Know   **Want to Know**
1 kg : 2.2 lb :: x kg : 122 lb
$(1 \times 122) = (2.2 \times x)$; $122 = 2.2x$; $122/2.2 = x$; $x = 55.45$ kg; round off to tenths: 55.5 kg
Proof: $1 \times 122 = 122$; $2.2 \times 55.45 = 121.99$ (rounds to 122)

Example 3: You have an injectable solution that is 50 mg strength. How many micrograms are in 50 mg?

Equivalent: 1 mg = 1000 mcg

Know   **Want to Know**
1 mg : 1000 mcg :: 50 mg : x mcg
$(1 \times x) = (1000 \times 50)$; $1x = 50,000$; $x = 50,000$; therefore, 50 mg = 50,000 mcg
Proof: $1 \times 50,000 = 50,000$; $1000 \times 50 = 50,000$

Example 4: An elixir is ordered as follows: "Give 2 tsp twice a day." How many millilitres would you give?

Equivalent: 1 tsp = 5 mL

Know   ***Want to Know***
1 tsp : 5 mL :: 2 tsp : x mL
$(1 \times x) = (5 \times 2)$; $1x = 10$; $x = 10$ mL
Proof: $1 \times 10 = 10$; $5 \times 2 = 10$; $10 = 10$
So, give 10 mL to equal 2 tsp.

Example 5: You have an injection that delivers 75 μg (mcg). How many milligrams does it deliver?

Equivalent: 1 mg = 1000 mcg

Know   ***Want to Know***
1 mg : 1000 mcg :: x mg : 75 mcg
$(1 \times 75) = (1000 \times x)$; $75 = 1000x$; $x = 75/1000$; $x = 0.075$
So, 75 mcg = 0.075 mg. *(Do not forget the leading zero!)*
Proof: $1 \times 75 = 75$; $1000 \times 0.075 = 75$; $75 = 75$

PRACTICE PROBLEMS

Calculate the following conversions.

1. 600 mg   = _____ mcg   10. 500 mL   = _____ L
2. 1500 mg   = _____ mcg   11. 90 mg   = _____ g
3. 5000 mcg = _____ mg   12. 4 tsp   = _____ mL
4. 5 g   = _____ mg   13. 60 mL   = _____ tsp
5. 2.5 g   = _____ mg   14. 90 mL   = _____ tbsp
6. 900 mg   = _____ g   15. 90 kg   = _____ lb
7. 8 kg   = _____ g   16. 150 lb   = _____ kg
8. 750 mL   = _____ L   17. 11 kg   = _____ lb
9. 975 L   = _____ mL

SECTION II: CALCULATING ORAL DOSES

To calculate oral dosages of medications, use the same ratio and proportion procedures described in Section I. Label all terms, and check your answers by proving them.

The first step in doing medication dosage calculation problems is examining the order and the medication on hand. The units for both the order and the medicine on hand MUST be the same units (e.g., mg, mL). If they are not the same, then a conversion must first be done to change the ordered dose to the same units as the medication on hand.

Remember these rules:

- NEVER substitute one form of a medication for another, even if the dosage amount is the same. Parenteral forms of oral drugs are much stronger, and the resulting effects might be dangerous.
- Do not forget to place a zero in front of a decimal point (e.g., 0.75 mg). It reminds you that the number is a decimal, not a whole number.
- Are the medication ordered and the medication on hand in the same units? If not, convert the drug ordered to the units of the drug on hand.

- Place what you have on hand (what you know)—information from the label—on the LEFT side of the equation.
- Place what is ordered (what you want to know) on the RIGHT side of the equation.
- Solve the equation as described in Section I.
- ALWAYS label the units of your answer (tablets, capsules, mL, etc.).

Example 1: The prescription reads, "Give 500 mg PO." The unit dose is 250 mg/tablet. How many tablets will you give?

Ordered: 500 mg   **Unit dose:** 250 mg/tablet
NOTE: Units match (mg).

Know   *Want to Know*
250 mg : 1 tablet :: 500 mg : x tablet
$(250 \times x) = (1 \times 500)$; $250x = 500$; $x = 500/250 = 2$
Answer: Give 2 tablets.
Proof: $250 \times 2 = 500$; $1 \times 500 = 500$; $500 = 500$

Example 2: The order is to give 175 mg. The tablets on hand are 350-mg scored tablets. How many tablets will you give?

Ordered: 175 mg   **Unit dose:** 350 mg/tablet
NOTE: Units match (mg).

Know   *Want to Know*
350 mg : 1 tablet :: 175 mg : x tablet
$(350 \times x) = (1 \times 175)$; $350x = 175$; $x = 175/350 = 0.5$
Answer: Give 0.5 tablet (one-half of the scored tablet).
Proof: $350 \times 0.5 = 175$; $1 \times 175 = 175$; $175 = 175$

Example 3: You are asked to administer 100 mg of a drug. You have 0.05-g tablets on hand. How many tablets will you give?

Ordered: 100 mg   **Unit dose:** 0.05 g/tablet
NOTE: Units do not match (mg and g).

First: Calculate: 100 mg = x g (Equivalent: 1 g = 1000 mg)

Know   *Want to Know*
1 g : 1000 mg :: x g : 100 mg
$(1 \times 100) = (1000 \times x)$; $100 = 1000x$; $x = 100/1000 = 0.1$
100 mg = 0.1 g
Now that you have the ordered dose and the dose on hand in the same units, you can complete the problem.
Ordered: 0.1 g (100 mg)   **Unit dose:** 0.05 g/tablet

Know   *Want to Know*
0.05 g : 1 tablet :: 0.1 g : x tablet
$(0.05 \times x) = (1 \times 0.1)$; $0.05x = 0.1$; $x = 0.1/0.05 = 2$
Answer: Give 2 tablets.
Proof: $0.05 \times 2 = 0.1$; $1 \times 0.1 = 0.1$; $0.1 = 0.1$

Example 4: You are instructed to give 0.5 g of a drug. You have 250-mg tablets on hand. How many tablets will you give?

Ordered: 0.5 g **Unit dose:** 250 mg/tablet
NOTE: Units do not match (g and mg).

First: Calculate: 0.5 g = x mg (Equivalent: 1 g = 1000 mg)

Know *Want to Know*
1 g : 1000 mg :: 0.5 g : x mg
$(1 \times x) = (1000 \times 0.5)$; $1x = 500$; $x = 500$
0.5 g = 500 mg
Now that you have the ordered dose and the dose on hand in the same units, you can complete the problem.
Ordered: 500 mg (0.5 g) **Unit dose:** 250 mg/tablet

Know *Want to Know*
250 mg : 1 tablet :: 500 mg : x tablet
$(250 \times x) = (1 \times 500)$; $250x = 500$; $x = 500/250 = 2$
Answer: Give 2 tablets.
Proof: $250 \times 2 = 500$; $1 \times 500 = 500$; $500 = 500$

Example 5: You are to administer 200 mg of guaifenesin syrup. You have a bottle labelled 100 mg/5 mL. How many mL will you give?

Ordered: 200 mg **Unit dose:** 100 mg/5 mL
NOTE: Units match (mg).

Know *Want to Know*
100 mg : 5 mL :: 200 mg : x mL
$(100 \times x) = (5 \times 200)$; $100x = 1000$; $x = 1000/100 = 10$
Answer: Give 10 mL.
Proof: $100 \times 10 = 1000$; $5 \times 200 = 1000$; $1000 = 1000$

PRACTICE PROBLEMS

1. Dose ordered: ascorbic acid 0.5 g PO
   Dose on hand: 500-mg tablets
   How many tablets will you give? _____

2. Dose ordered: digoxin 0.5 mg PO
   Dose on hand: 250-mcg tablets
   How many tablets will you give? _____

3. Dose ordered: sulfisoxazole 0.25 g PO
   Dose on hand: 500-mg tablets
   How many tablets will you give? _____

4. Dose ordered: diphenhydramine elixir 50 mg PO
   Dose on hand: elixir 12.5 mg/5 mL
   How many millilitres will you give? _____

5. Dose ordered: cefaclor 0.1 g PO
   Dose on hand: liquid 125 mg/5 mL
   How many millilitres will you give? _____

6. Dose ordered: zidovudine 0.3 g PO
   Dose on hand: 100-mg tablets
   How many tablets will you give? _____

7. Dose ordered: potassium chloride elixir 30 mEq PO
   Dose on hand: 20 mEq/15 mL
   How many millilitres will you give? _____

8. Dose ordered: pentobarbital 0.15 g PO
   Dose on hand: 50-mg capsules
   How many capsules will you give? _____

9. Dose ordered: levodopa 2 g PO
   Dose on hand: 500-mg tablets
   How many tablets will you give? _____

SECTION III: RECONSTITUTING MEDICATIONS

Many medications come in powder or crystal form and must be reconstituted by the addition of a diluent to create a liquid form. Many parenteral medications must be reconstituted before administration. Instructions for dissolving medications can be found in the literature that accompanies the medication or on the medication label. Most of the time, medications that need to be reconstituted are in delivery systems that match 50- or 100-mL IV bags, and reconstitution occurs as the nurse prepares the medication for use. However, there are still instances where the nurse may be required to reconstitute a drug and then draw up the proper dose for parenteral use. These examples are for those instances.

For example, the instructions may read:

Add 1.2 mL normal saline to make 2 mL of reconstituted solution that yields 100 mg/mL.

This tells the user that the medication takes up 0.8 mL of space: 1.2 mL + 0.8 mL = 2 mL of medication solution. The label of the medication container will tell the user how many units, grams, milligrams, or micrograms are in each millilitre of the reconstituted drug. In this example, the dose on hand, after reconstitution, is 100 mg/mL.

Remember these rules:
- Read all instructions for reconstitution before doing anything! Be sure to ask a pharmacist if you have any questions.
- When reconstituting medications, be certain to use the exact **type** of diluent, and add the exact **amount** of diluent as directed. Substitutions or inaccurate amounts of diluent can inactivate the medication or alter the concentration, thus altering the dose received by the patient.
- If the vial is a multiple-dose vial, the nurse who reconstitutes the medication must put the date, time, amount of diluent used, and the nurse's initials on the label.
- Many solutions are unstable after being reconstituted. Be sure to follow the directions on the label for proper storage of reconstituted medications.
- Make note of the time limit or expiration date for the reconstituted medication. Do not use the medication after it has expired.
- Ratio solutions indicate the number of grams of the medication per total millilitres of solution. For example, a medication that is designated 1:1000 has 1 g of medication per 1000 mL of solution.

In order to avoid overdosing, it is essential that the nurse chooses the correct ratio solution!
- Percentage (%) solutions indicate the number of grams of the medication per 100 mL of solution. For example, a medication that is designated 10% has 10 g of drug per 100 mL of solution.
- COMPARE: "1:1000" indicates 1 g per 1000 mL
              "10%" indicates 10 g per 100 mL

As you calculate parenteral dosages:
- If the amount is greater than 1 mL, round x (the amount to be given) to tenths and use a 3-mL syringe to measure it.
- Small (less than 0.5 mL, or child) dosages should be rounded to hundredths and measured in a tuberculin syringe. The tuberculin syringe is calibrated in 0.01-mL increments.
- THINK! For adults, the maximum volume of an intramuscular (IM) injection is usually 3 mL. Sometimes the dose might have to be given in two divided doses; for example, a dose of 4 mL IM would usually be divided into two 2-mL doses. However, if your calculations yield an unusual number, such as 10 mL IM, look over your calculation and repeat your math! Double-check your calculations with a peer.

Always remember to note the route ordered. IM doses and IV doses are NOT always the same amount, and the drug formulations may differ; confusing the route can have fatal results.

Example 1: You receive an order for morphine 10 mg IM. The medication vial reads 8 mg/mL.

How much morphine would you give?
Does this medication require reconstitution?
Would you use a 3-mL or a tuberculin syringe to measure this drug?
Ordered: 10 mg   **Unit dose:** 8 mg/mL

Know   *Want to Know*
8 mg : 1 mL :: 10 mg : x mL
$(8 \times x) = (1 \times 10)$; $8x = 10$; $x = 10/8 = 1.25$, rounded to 1.3
Answer: 1.3 mL measured in a 3-mL syringe. This medication does not require reconstitution.
Proof: $8 \times 1.3 = 10.4$ (rounds to 10); $1 \times 10 = 10$

Example 2: The ordered dose is cloxacillin sodium 500 mg IV. The medication label reads as shown below:

> 500 mg CLOXACILLIN SODIUM FOR INJECTION
> For IM or IV use
> Add 2.7 mL sterile water for injection.
> Each 1.5 mL contains 250 mg cloxacillin.

How much cloxacillin would you give?
Does this medication require reconstitution?
Would you use a 3-mL or a tuberculin syringe to measure this drug?
Ordered: 500 mg   **Unit dose:** 250 mg/1.5 mL

Know   *Want to Know*
250 mg : 1.5 mL :: 500 mg : x mL
$(250 \times x) = (1.5 \times 500)$; $250x = 750$; $x = 750/250 = 3$
Answer: 3 mL measured in a 3-mL syringe. Reconstitute by adding 2.7 mL sterile water to the vial.
Proof: $250 \times 3 = 750$; $1.5 \times 500 = 750$; $750 = 750$

Example 3: You receive an order for penicillin G potassium 400,000 units IM. The medication label reads as shown below:

> ONE MILLION UNITS
> Penicillin G Potassium
> Use sterile saline as diluent as follows:
> Add   Units per mL reconstituted solution
> 18.2 mL   250,000
> 8.2 mL   500,000
> 3.2 mL   1,000,000

Which dilution would you choose for the ordered dose?
How much penicillin G potassium would you give?
Would you use a 3-mL or a tuberculin syringe to measure this drug?
Ordered: 400,000 units   **Unit dose:** Choosing the 8.2 diluent amount, the unit dose is 500,000/mL.

Know   *Want to Know*
500,000 units : 1 mL :: 400,000 : x mL
$(500,000 \times x) = (1 \times 400,000)$; $500,000x = 400,000$; $x = 400,000/500,000 = 0.8$
Answer: 0.8 mL measured in either a 3-mL or tuberculin syringe
Proof: $500,000 \times 0.8 = 400,000$; $1 \times 400,000 = 400,000$; $400,000 = 400,000$

NOTE: Choose the concentration that is close to the ordered dose. Choosing the 8.2 diluent amount allows for the injection amount to be small yet easily measured. If you had chosen the 18.2 diluent amount, the injection would have been 1.6 mL; choosing the 3.2 diluent would have made the injection amount very small (0.04 mL).

Example 4: You receive an order for epinephrine 0.6 mg SC. The medication label reads as shown below:

> 1 mL ampule
> Epinephrine 1:1000
> For SC or IM use

What is the dose on hand?
How much epinephrine would you give?
Would you use a 3-mL or a tuberculin syringe to measure the drug?
First: Figure the dose on hand.
1:1000 = 1 g in 1000 mL = 1000 mg in 1000 mL = **1 mg in 1 mL**

Then complete the problem:
Ordered: 0.6 mg   **Unit dose:** 1 mg/mL

Know   *Want to Know*
1 mg : 1 mL :: 0.6 mg : x mL
$(1 \times x) = (1 \times 0.6)$; $1x = 0.6$; $x = 0.6$
Answer: 0.6 mL measured in either a 3-mL or tuberculin syringe.
Proof: $1 \times 0.6 = 0.6$; $1 \times 0.6 = 0.6$; $0.6 = 0.6$

Example 5: Magnesium sulfate 5 g IV over 3 hours is the dosage ordered. The medication label reads as shown below:

> 10 mL vial
> Magnesium sulfate 10%
> For IM or IV use

What is the dose on hand?
How much magnesium sulfate would you give?
First: Figure the dose on hand.
10% = 10 g in 100 mL = **0.1 g per 1 mL**

Then complete the problem:
Ordered: 5 g **Unit dose:** 0.1 g/mL

Know   *Want to Know*
0.1 g : 1 mL :: 5 g : x mL
$(0.1 \times x) = (1 \times 5)$; $0.1x = 5$; $x = 5/0.1$; $x = 50$
Answer: 50 mL
Proof: $0.1 \times 50 = 5$; $1 \times 5 = 5$; $5 = 5$

PRACTICE PROBLEMS

1. Dose ordered: thiamine 200 mg
   On hand: 10-mL vial, 100 mg/mL
   How much will you give? _____

2. Dose ordered: gentamicin 60 mg IM
   On hand: 40 mg/mL
   How much will you give? _____

3. Dose ordered: heparin 8000 units SC
   On hand: 1-mL vial, 10,000 units/mL
   How much will you give? _____

4. Dose ordered: methicillin 750 mg IV
   On hand: 1-g vial
   Instructions for reconstitution: Add 1.5 mL sterile water. Reconstituted solution will contain approximately 500 mg methicillin solution per mL.
   How much will you give? _____

5. Dose ordered: ampicillin 500 mg IV
   On hand: 1-g vial
   Instructions for reconstitution: Add 66 mL sterile water. Reconstituted solution will contain 125 mg/5 mL.
   How much will you give? _____

6. Dose ordered: penicillin G potassium 300,000 units IM
   On hand: 1,000,000-unit vial
   Instructions for reconstitution: Using only sterile water, add 9.6 mL to provide 100,000 units/mL, or 4.6 mL to provide 200,000 units/mL. Which concentration would you choose for this dose? _____
   How much will you give? _____

7. Dose ordered: epinephrine 750 mcg SC
   On hand: 1:1000
   How much will you give? _____

8. Dose ordered: isoproterol hydrochloride 0.2 mg
   On hand: 1:5000
   How much will you give? _____

9. Dose ordered: calcium gluconate 900 mg
   On hand: calcium gluconate 10%, 100-mg/mL vial
   How much will you give? _____

10. Dose ordered: magnesium sulfate 4 g
    On hand: magnesium sulfate 50%, 10-mL vial
    How much will you give? _____

SECTION IV: CHILD CALCULATIONS

Doses used in children must differ from those used in adults. The most common method for calculating doses for children is weight based (i.e., mg/kg). In some cases, dosages may be calculated using body surface area (BSA) calculations.

Body Surface Area (BSA) Calculations

The BSA is a common method used to calculate therapeutic children's dosages. It requires the use of a chart, called a West nomogram (see Figure 3-1 on p. 47 in the textbook), that converts weight to square metres (m^2) of BSA. The average adult is assumed to weigh 63.5 kg (140 lb) and have a BSA of $1.73 m^2$. The BSA may be used to calculate the child dose of certain medications.

- For a child of normal height and weight, find the BSA in square metres for that weight on the shaded area of the nomogram chart.
  Example: Using Figure 3-1 in your text, find the BSA for a child who weighs 18.1 kg (25 lb) and is 95 cm (38 inches) tall (normal weight for her height). According to the nomogram, the BSA for 40 lb is $0.74 m^2$.

- For a child who is underweight or overweight, the BSA is indicated at the point where a straight line connecting the height and weight intersects the unshaded surface area (SA) column.
  Example: Using Figure 3-1, find the BSA for a child who weighs 11.4 kg (25 lb) and has a height of 75 cm (30 inches) (underweight). According to the nomogram, the BSA for this child is $0.51 m^2$.

There are two types of BSA problems.

1. The first type involves medications for which the literature provides recommended dosages in square metres.

   STEP 1: Check the order, and look up the recommended dose.
   The order is for 15 mg PO.
   The literature states that $40 mg/m^2$ is safe for children.

   STEP 2: Determine the child's height and weight. Then consult the appropriate nomogram to obtain the BSA in square metres. This child weighs 10 kg (22 lb) and has a normal height of 70 cm. The BSA is approximately $0.46 m^2$.

   STEP 3: Calculate the recommended mg/m^2 dose (from the literature), using ratio and proportion. Then, for a safety check, compare it with the dose ordered.
   For this calculation, what you *know* is the literature's recommendation ($40 mg/m^2$). What you *want to know* is the milligrams per the child's BSA (which is $0.46 m^2$).

Know **Want to Know**
40 mg : 1 m² :: x mg : 0.46 m²
(40 × 0.46) = (1 × x); 18.4 = 1x; x = 18.4 (Child doses are rounded to tenths place; *do not* round to whole numbers.)
Answer: 18.4 mg is the safe dose limit.
Decision: The order for 15 mg is safe.

Practice:
The medication ordered is 100 mg.

STEP 1: The literature recommends 50 mg/m² for children.

STEP 2: The child weighs 4.5 kg (10 lb) and has a normal height for his weight. The BSA is 0.27 m².

STEP 3: Calculate the dose for this child's BSA:

Know **Want to Know**
50 mg : 1 m² :: x mg : 0.27 m²
(50 × 0.27) = (1 × x); 13.5 = 1x; x = 13.5 (Child doses are rounded to tenths place; *do not* round to whole numbers.)
Answer: 13.5 mg is the safe dose limit.
Decision: The order for 15 mg exceeds the safe dose limit and therefore is NOT safe. Notify the physician.

2. The second type of BSA involves situations when a recommended dose is cited in the literature for adults but not for children.

   STEP 1: Determine the BSA (in square metres) of the child by dividing the adult dose by 1.73 m² (the average adult's BSA).

   STEP 2: Multiply the result by the average adult dose.

$$\frac{\text{child's BSA (m}^2)}{\text{average adult's BSA (m}^2)} \times \text{average adult dose of drug} = \text{estimated child dose}$$

   Example: A 2.7-kg (6-lb) child has a BSA of 0.20 m², and the average adult dose of a drug is 300 mg. What would be the estimated safe dose for a child?

$$\frac{0.20 \, \text{m}^2}{1.73 \, \text{m}^2} \times 300 \, \text{mg} = 34.68 \, \text{mg}$$

   Answer: 34.7 mg is the estimated safe dose for this child. (Round to tenths place for child doses.)

Practice:
The average adult dose for a medication is 20 mg. The child has a BSA of 0.6 m².
What would be the estimated safe dose for a child?

$$\frac{0.6 \, \text{m}^2}{1.73 \, \text{m}^2} \times 20 \, \text{mg} = 6.94 \, \text{mg}$$

Answer: 6.9 mg is the estimated safe dose for this child. (Round to tenths place for child doses.)

Weight-Based Calculations

When calculating the proper dose according to weight, **STEP 1** involves changing the weight from pounds to kilograms (if necessary).

- Be careful when converting ounces and pounds to kilograms. First, ounces must be converted to part of a pound (by dividing the ounces by 16). Remember, 16 ounces = 1 pound. Therefore, 8 oz does not convert to 0.8 lb! Convert 8 ounces to pounds by dividing by 16: 8/16 = 0.5; 8 oz = 0.5 lb.
- Once you have converted ounces to pounds, add the ounces to the pounds. For example, 10 lb 8 oz would equal 10.5 lb. You are now ready to convert pounds to kilograms.
- Remember, 1 kg = 2.2 lb. To convert 10.5 lb to kilograms, divide the pounds by 2.2. 1 kg : 2.2 lb :: x kg : 10.5 lb; (1 × 10.5) = (2.2 × x); 10.5 = 2.2x; x = 10.5/2.2 = 4.8 kg (rounded to tenths)
- DO NOT round child weights to whole numbers!

Once you have converted the child's weight to kilograms, you are ready for STEP 2.

STEP 2 involves calculating the therapeutic dosage ranges for a child, based on his or her weight. The nurse uses the child's weight (in kilograms) to calculate the low and high acceptable doses for that medication. This will give a range of dosages that this child could receive for this medication.

STEP 3 involves THINKING and comparing the ordered dose with the therapeutic dosage range that was calculated for that child. If the ordered dose is under or over the calculated therapeutic dosage range, then do not give the medication, and notify the physician.

- **STEP 1:** Convert the child's weight from pounds to kilograms.

- **STEP 2:** Calculate the therapeutic dose range (low and high).

- **STEP 3:** (1) Is the ordered dose safe (does not exceed the dosage range)?
  (2) Is the ordered dose therapeutic (falling within the recommended dosage range, not too low)?

Example 1: The ordered dose is 50 mg of acetaminophen. The infant weighs 15 lb. The therapeutic dosage range for acetaminophen is 10 to 15 mg/kg/dose.

STEP 1: Convert pounds to kilograms by dividing 15 by 2.2.
15/2.2 = 6.82; 15 lb = 6.8 kg (Round child weights to tenths, not to whole numbers.)

STEP 2: Calculate the therapeutic dosage range for this infant based on his weight.
Low dose: 10 mg/kg/dose × 6.8 kg = 68 mg/dose (note that the "kg" cancels out).
High dose: 15 mg/kg/dose × 6.8 kg = 102 mg/dose (note that the "kg" cancels out).
The therapeutic dosage range for this infant is 68 to 102 mg/dose for acetaminophen.

STEP 3: Compare the ordered dose with the therapeutic dosage range calculated in STEP 2.
Answer: The ordered dose of 50 mg is not therapeutic because it falls under the low recommended dose.

If the doctor orders 110 mg of acetaminophen for this infant, would that be a safe and therapeutic dose?

Answer: No, it would be neither safe nor therapeutic because it is higher than 102 mg.

Example 2: The ordered dose is amoxicillin 275 mg q8h PO. The child weighs 35 lb. The therapeutic dosage range for amoxicillin is 20 to 40 mg/kg/24 hr.

STEP 1: Convert pounds to kilograms by dividing 35 by 2.2.
35/2.2 = 15.9; 35 lb = 15.9 kg

STEP 2: Calculate the therapeutic dosage range for this child based on his weight.
Low dose: 20 mg/kg/24 hr × 15.9 kg = 318 mg/24 hr
High dose: 40 mg/kg/24 hr × 15.9 kg = 636 mg/24 hr

NOTE: These ranges are for 24 hours! The dosage is every 8 hours, so dividing 24 hours by 8 tells us that there will be 3 doses within 24 hours. To figure out the single dosage for the low and high ranges, divide each 24-hour dose by 3:
318 mg/24 hr divided by 3 doses = 106 mg/dose
636 mg/24 hr divided by 3 doses = 212 mg/dose
Answer: The safe range for a single dose of amoxicillin for this child is 106 to 212 mg/dose.

(An alternate way to figure a single dose is to calculate the amount of medication the ordered dose would provide in 24 hours. In this example, knowing there are three doses given every 8 hours in a 24-hour period, multiplying the dose ordered by 3 would yield the ordered dose for 24 hours: 275 mg × 3 doses = 825 mg/24 hr.)

STEP 3: Is the ordered dose of 275 mg therapeutic for this child?
Answer: No, the ordered dose of 275 mg exceeds the therapeutic dosage range for this child. Consult the physician. (Note also that the calculated 24-hour dose of 825 mg/24 hr exceeds the high range of 636 mg/24 hr calculated for this child.)

Many pediatric medications come in several concentrations. It is ESSENTIAL to use the correct concentration of medication to ensure accurate dosage and prevent accidental underdosage or overdosage.

Example: Acetaminophen comes in many forms, including the following:
Drops, 80 mg/mL
Syrup, 80 or 120 or 160 mg/5 mL
Liquid oral solution, 32 or 80 or 160 mg/mL
Liquid suspension, 160 mg/5 mL
Chewable tablets, 80 or 160 mg
Tablets, 80 or 325 or 500 mg
Tablets, extended-release, 650 mg
Suppositories, 120 mg, 160 mg, 125 mg, 325 mg, or 650 mg

A 4-month-old infant weighs 13 lb and has a fever of 38.6°C. What would be the therapeutic dosage range of acetaminophen this infant could receive?

STEP 1: 13 lb = 5.9 kg

STEP 2: Low dose: 10 mg/kg/dose × 5.9 = 59 mg/dose
High dose: 15 mg/kg/dose × 5.9 = 88.5 mg/dose
Answer: The therapeutic dosage range for this infant is 59 to 88.5 mg/dose.
Referring to the forms of acetaminophen listed above, which form would you choose if this infant was to receive an 80-mg dose?
Answer: Choose the drops or suspension, 80 mg/mL, and administer 1 mL with a calibrated oral syringe or dropper.

STEP 3: Is the ordered dose of 60 mg therapeutic for this infant?
Answer: Yes, the 60 mg dose falls within the 59 to 88.5 mg/dose range for this infant.

Why choose the drops? Remember, you are giving medication to an infant. The infant cannot take tablets; suppositories are not the first choice unless the infant cannot take oral medications, and rectal doses may be a little higher than oral doses. You should choose the medication form that is manufactured for infants and the form that will deliver the dose in an amount that is easily measured yet not too much for the infant to swallow. For example, if you chose the elixir or liquid suspension, 160 mg/5 mL, then you would need to give 2.5 mL. The 0.6 mL would be easier to administer to an infant. **NOTE:** Most liquid medication packages for infants and children have specific instructions for dosing and include the specific dropper to use for measuring liquids.

PRACTICE PROBLEMS

1. Your 6-year-old patient weighs 40 lb. Morphine sulfate via continuous infusion is ordered at 1 mg/hr. The therapeutic dosage range for continuous intravenous infusion is 0.025 to 2.6 mg/kg/hr.
   a. What are the low and high doses for this child? _____
   b. Is the ordered dose within a safe and therapeutic range? _____

2. A 5-year-old weighs 33 lb. Ibuprofen is ordered at 120 mg PO q8h. The therapeutic dosage range is 5 to 10 mg/kg/dose q6h to q8h, and the maximum dose is 40 mg/kg/24 hr.
   a. What are the low and high doses for this child? _____
   b. What is the maximum amount this child can receive in 24 hours? _____
   c. Is the ordered dose within a safe and therapeutic range? _____

3. A 10-year-old patient weighs 70 lb. Ceftazidine is ordered at 1.7 g q8h IV. The therapeutic dosage range is 100 to 150 mg/kg/24 h (divided q8h IV).
   a. What are the low and high doses for this child in 24 hours? _____
   b. What are the low and high doses for this child per individual dose? _____
   c. Is the ordered dose within a safe and therapeutic range? _____

4. Your patient weighs 15 lb. The medication ordered is 150 mcg bid. The therapeutic dosage range of the medication is 0.02 to 0.05 mg/kg/day.
   a. What are the low and high doses for this child in 24 hours? _____
   b. What are the low and high doses for this child per individual dose? _____
   c. Is the ordered dose within a safe and therapeutic range? _____

5. A child weighs 34 lb. The medication ordered is 30 mg IM preoperatively. The therapeutic dosage range is 1 to 2.2 mg/kg.
   a. What are the low and high doses for this child per individual dose? _____
   b. Is the ordered dose within a safe and therapeutic range? _____

6. For a child weighing 50 lb, medication is ordered at 0.2 mg daily IV. The therapeutic dosage range is 4 to 5 mcg/kg/day.
   a. What are the low and high doses for this child per individual dose? _____
   b. Is the ordered dose within a safe and therapeutic range? _____

SECTION V: BASIC INTRAVENOUS CALCULATIONS

Intravenous (IV) fluids and medications are given over a designated period of time. For instance, the order may read:

Give 1000 mL normal saline over 8 hours IV.

For IVs that infuse with an infusion pump, the rate in millilitres per hour (mL/hr) is calculated.
For IVs that infuse by gravity, the rate at which an IV is given is measured in terms of *drops per minute* (gtt/min).

To calculate mL/hr and gtt/min, consider what the order contains and what equipment is used. In order to calculate drops per minute, it is important to know the drop factor of the IV tubing. The size of the drops delivered per millilitre can vary with different types of tubing. The drop factor of a certain tubing set is printed on the packaging label.
Adding to the above order:

The drop factor for the IV tubing is 15 gtt/mL.

The order now reads:

Give 1000 mL normal saline over 8 hours IV. The drop factor is 15 gtt/mL.

STEP 1: Calculate millilitres per hour.

We *know* that 1000 mL is to infuse over 8 hours. We *want to know* how much is to infuse over 1 hour. Set up the equation:

Know   *Want to Know*

1000 mL : 8 hours :: x mL : 1 hour

$(1000 \times 1) = (8 \times x)$; $1000 = 8x$; $x = 8/1000$; $x = 125$ mL/hr

Rate: To give 1000 mL normal saline over 8 hours, give 125 mL/hr for 8 hours.

A quick way to determine the hourly rate is to divide the TOTAL VOLUME by the TOTAL TIME (if the time is in hours): 1000 mL × 8 hours = 125 mL/hr.

STEP 2: Calculate the drops per minute.

To set up a gravity IV drip, further calculations are needed. To ensure the proper rate, one must count the drops per minute (gtt/min).

We know the rate is 125 mL/hr and the drop factor is 15 gtt/mL. Since we need to change from *hours* to *minutes*, another equivalent we will need is 60 minutes = 1 hour.

When the millilitres per hour are known, the formula for calculating the drops per minute is as follows:

$$\frac{\text{drop factor}}{\text{time (min)}} \times \text{hourly rate (mL/hr)} = \text{gtt/min}$$

Plugging in what we know:

$$\frac{15 \text{ gtt/mL}^{*}}{60 \text{ min/hr}} \times 125/\text{hr} = x \text{ gtt/min}$$

*To make it easier to calculate, reduce the 15/60 fraction to 1/4 before multiplying by 125.

$1/4 \times 125 = 125/4 = 31.25$ (Round mL/hr to whole numbers.)

Answer: 31 gtt/min for a gravity drip

Points to remember:

- The drop factor varies per IV tubing set manufacturer. It can range from 10 to 60 gtt/min.
- Infusion sets that deliver 60 gtt/min are called *microdrips*.
- STEP 1: To calculate millilitres per hour, divide the TOTAL VOLUME by the TOTAL TIME (in hours).
- STEP 2: To calculate drops per minute when the hourly rate is known, use the formula:

$$\frac{\text{drop factor (gtt/mL)}}{\text{time (min)}} \times \text{hourly rate (mL/hr)} = \text{gtt/min}$$

- THINK! If you are using an infusion pump, you need to calculate milliliters per hour.
- THINK! Round off your answer to the nearest whole number. You cannot count a partial drop! Also, IV electronic infusion pumps will usually use the nearest whole number in millilitres. (Exceptions to this may occur in pediatric settings.)

Example 1: The order reads "200 mL to be infused for 1 hour." If the drop factor is 15 gtt/mL, how many gtt/min will be given?

Start at STEP 1 or STEP 2?

Start at

STEP 1: Calculate millilitres per hour.

STEP 1: Divide the total volume by the total time (in hours).

200 mL over 1 hour = 200 mL/hr.

STEP 2: Calculate the drop per minute, using the formula given above:

$$\frac{\text{drop factor}}{\text{time (min)}} \times \text{hourly rate} = 15/60 \times 200 = 1/4 \times 200 = 50$$

Answer: 50 gtt/min

Example 2: The order is for 1000 mL to infuse at 150 mL/hr. The drop factor is 20 gtt/mL. How many drops per minute will be given?
Start at STEP 1 or STEP 2?
Start at STEP 2. The hourly rate, 150 mL/hr, has been given.
STEP 2: Calculate the drops per minute:

$$\frac{\text{drop factor}}{\text{time (min)}} \times \text{hourly rate} = 20/60 \times 150 = 1/3 \times 150 = 50$$

Answer: 50 gtt/min

Example 3: You receive an order for 200 mL to be infused for 90 minutes. You have a microdrip set (60 gtt/mL). How many drops per minute will be given?
Start at STEP 1 or STEP 2?
Start at STEP 1. Calculate the hourly rate. Remember, 60 minutes = 1 hour.
STEP 1:

Know   ***Want to Know***
200 mL : 90 min :: *x* mL : 60 min
(200 × 60) = (90 × *x*); 12,000 = 90*x*; *x* = 12,000/90 *x* = 133.33
Rate: 133 mL/hr (Round to nearest whole number.)
STEP 2: Calculate the drops per minute:

$$\frac{\text{drop factor}}{\text{time (min)}} \times \text{hourly rate} = 60/60 \times 133 = 1 \times 133 = 133$$

Answer: 133 gtt/min
Short-cut: For microdrips, when the drip factor is 60 and the time is 60 minutes, the "60s" cancel out to "1," and the result is that the ordered milliliters per hour (mL/hr) equals the drop per minute (gtt/min).

PRACTICE PROBLEMS

Calculate the following, and prove your answers.

1. Give 1000 mL lactated Ringer's solution over 6 hours. The drop factor is 15 gtt/mL.
   Start at STEP 1 or STEP 2?
   a. mL/hr: _____
   b. gtt/min: _____

2. Infuse 600 mL blood over 3 hours. The blood administration set has a drop factor of 10 gtt/mL.
   Start at STEP 1 or STEP 2
   a. mL/hr: _____
   b. gtt/min: _____

3. Infuse 1000 mL normal saline over 12 hours, using tubing with a drop factor of 15 gtt/mL.
   Start at STEP 1 or STEP 2?
   a. mL/hr: _____
   b. gtt/min: _____

4. Infuse 200 mL D5NS over 2 hours, using a microdrip set.
   Start at STEP 1 or STEP 2?
   a. mL/hr: _____
   b. gtt/min: _____
   c. What is the drop factor? _____

5. Infuse D5W at 75 mL/hr. The drop factor is 10 gtt/mL.
   Start at STEP 1 or STEP 2?
   gtt/min: _____

6. Infuse D5W at 75 mL/hr. The drop factor is 15 gtt/mL.
   Start at STEP 1 or STEP 2?
   gtt/min: _____

7. Infuse D5W at 75 mL/hr. The drop factor is 15 gtt/mL.
   Start at STEP 1 or STEP 2?
   gtt/min: _____

8. After looking at your answers for questions 5, 6, and 7, what observation can you make about the relationship between the drop factor and the resulting drops per minute?

9. Give 50 mL of an antibiotic over 30 minutes. You will be using an infusion pump.
Start at STEP 1 or STEP 2?
   a. mL/hr: _____
   b. gtt/min: _____

c. Do you need to calculate both millilitres per hour and drops per minute for this situation? _____

10. Infuse 500 mL normal saline over 4 hours, using tubing with a drop factor of 60 gtt/mL.
Start at STEP 1 or STEP 2?
   a. mL/hr: _____
   b. gtt/min: _____

REFERENCE

Health Canada (2009). Drug identification number (DIN). Retrieved December 15, 2009, from http://www.hc-sc.gc.ca/dhp-mps/prodpharma/activit/fs-fi/dinfs_fd-eng.php

PRACTICE QUIZ

Convert the following.

1. 750 mcg = _____ mg

2. 8 g = _____ mg

3. 250 lb = _____ kg

4. 75 kg = _____ lb

5. 3 tsp = _____ mL

Calculate the following, and prove your answers.

6. Dose ordered: indomethacin (oral suspension) 50 mg qid
   Dose on hand: oral suspension 25 mg/5 mL
   How much would you give per dose? _____

7. Dose ordered: procainamide 0.5 g q4h
   Dose on hand: 500-mg tablets
   How much would you give per dose? _____

8. Dose ordered: phenytoin 100 mg IV now
   Dose on hand: 5-mL ampules labelled "0mg/mL"
   How much would you give per dose? _____

9. Dose ordered: lidocaine 50 mg IV now
   Dose on hand: lidocaine 1% in 5-mL ampules
   How much would you give? _____

10. Dose ordered: epinephrine 0.25 mg SC now
    Dose on hand: epinephrine 1:1000 ampules
    How much would you give? _____

11. Dose ordered: heparin 15,000 units IV bolus
    Dose on hand: heparin 10,000 units/mL (5-mL vial)
    How much would you give? _____

12. Dose ordered: hydrochlorathiazide 1 mg/kg PO daily
    Child's weight: 22 lb
    Therapeutic dosage range: 2 mg/kg divided bid
    a. What is the safe and therapeutic range for this child? _____
    b. Is the ordered dose safe and therapeutic? _____

13. Ordered: Infuse normal saline 500 mL over 8 hours. The tubing drop factor is 15.
    a. What is the rate of the IV? _____
    b. What is the number of drops per minute? _____

14. Ordered: D51/2 normal saline to infuse at 50 mL/hr via an infusion pump.
    a. How will this be administered—as millilitres per hour or as drop per minute? _____
    b. What is the rate? _____

15. Ordered: 1000 mL D5W to infuse over 24 hours. The tubing drop factor is 60.
    a. What is the rate of the IV? _____
    b. What is the number of drops per minute? _____

16. Ordered: cefuroxime 500 mg IVPB q6h
    Dose on hand: cefuroxime powder for injection (see label)

> 750 mg vial
> CEFUROXIME
> Add 8 mL sterile water for injection.
> Solution will contain 90 mg/mL.

a. How much does this vial contain? _____
b. How much will you give for each dose? _____

17. Ordered: penicillin G 200,000 units IM qid
Dose on hand: penicillin G 5,000,000 units
The medication label reads as shown below:

FIVE MILLION UNITS multidose vial
Penicillin G
Use sterile saline as diluent as follows:
Add   Units per mL reconstituted solution
23 mL   200,000
18 mL   250,000
8 mL   500,000
3 mL   1,000,000

a. What concentration should you choose? _____

b. How much sterile saline should you add to the vial to obtain this concentration? _____

c. How much medication will you give? _____

d. How do you label the vial? _____

18. A child weighs 31 lb.
Dose ordered: ceftriaxone sodium 600 mg IV q12 h
Dose on hand: See label.
Maximum safe dose: up to 100 mg/kg/day in two divided doses

1 g
ceftriaxone sodium
DIRECTIONS: Add 9.6 mL sterile water for injection to equal 100 mg/mL.

a. How much would you give for this dose? _____

b. What is the maximum safe dose for this child (in 24 hours)? _____

c. What is the maximum safe dose for this child (per dose)? _____

d. Is the ordered dose within a safe and therapeutic range? _____

19. Dose ordered: digoxin 125 mcg daily
Dose on hand: pediatric elixir 0.05 mg/mL
How much would you give? _____

Answers

CHAPTER 1
Nursing Practice in Canada and Drug Therapy

Chapter Review/Critical Thinking and Application

1. a
2. d
3. c
4. b
5. a
6. b
7. S, O, O, O, S, S
8. Answers may vary slightly with each one but should include the following:
   - *Right drug (or right medication):* Compare drug orders and medication labels. Consider whether the drug is appropriate for that patient. Obtain information about the patient regarding past and present medical history, and obtain a thorough updated medication history, including over-the-counter (OTC) medications.
   - *Right dose:* Check the order and the label on the medication, and check for all of the 5 rights at least three times before administering the medication. Recheck the math calculations for dosages, and contact the physician when clarification is needed.
   - *Right time:* Assess for a conflict between the pharmacokinetic and pharmacodynamic properties of the drugs prescribed and the patient's lifestyle and likelihood of adherence.
   - *Right route:* Never assume the route for administration or change it; always check with the physician or prescriber.
   - *Right patient:* Check the patient's identity before administering a medication. Ask for the patient's name, and check the identification band or bracelet to confirm the patient's name, ID number, age, and allergies.
   - *Right reason:* Ensure that the drug ordered is being given for the right reason, necessitating prior knowledge of the drug's actions and adverse effects.
   - *Right documentation:* Ensure that documentation of the medication administration is done after the drug has been administered, not before; moreover, ensure that any unusual variances in time, dose, and drug reactions are properly recorded, as well as if the patient has refused the drug.
   - *Right evaluation (or right assessment):* Ensure that any special assessment requirements have been made prior to the drug administration, such as specific pulse rate and blood pressure readings, and laboratory results; moreover, ensure that appropriate monitoring of the patient has been done following drug administration and that follow-up measures are taken if the drug has not achieved its desired effect.
   - *Right patient education:* Ensure that the patient has been given proper explanation of the drug being given, the reason for its administration, and what to expect in terms of the drug's effects and possible adverse effects.
   - *Right to refuse:* Ensure that patients know they have a right to refuse the drug being administered and to inform them properly of the potential consequences of refusal.
9. a. Assessment
   b. Objective
   c. Subjective
   d. Analyze
   e. Goals
   f. Outcome criteria
   g. Implementation
   h. Evaluation

Case Study

1. See the discussion in Chapter 1, under Assessment. Important points include the following:
   - Use of prescription and over-the-counter medications

- Use of natural health products, including home remedies and vitamins
- Intake of alcohol, tobacco, and caffeine
- Current or prior use of illicit drugs
- Personal health history
- Family history
- Allergies

2. The medication order is missing the ROUTE of delivery and the DOSE amount. The nurse should contact the physician to clarify the incomplete order.

3. Again, the nurse should contact the physician and never change the medication route without an order.

4. After administering a drug, the nurse should evaluate the patient's response to the drug therapy. In this case, monitoring intake and output, monitoring vital signs, and observing for postural hypotension would be important.

CHAPTER 2
Pharmacological Principles

Chapter Review/Critical Thinking and Application

1. 1= c; 2 = d; 3 = a; 4 = b
2. c
3. b
4. d
5. a
6. c
7. b
8. h
9. i
10. f
11. g
12. a
13. d
14. e
15. c
16. Because muscles have a greater blood supply than the skin, drugs injected intramuscularly are typically absorbed more quickly than those injected subcutaneously. Absorption can be increased by applying heat to the injection site or by massaging it, which increases the blood flow to the area and thus enhances absorption.
17. This is an example of palliative therapy—drug therapy that is not curative but is intended to make the patient as comfortable as possible.

Case Study

1. Half-life is the time it takes for one half of the original amount of a drug in the body to be eliminated and is a measure of the rate at which drugs are excreted by the body. If the half-life is 2 hours, then in this example the drug level would be reduced as follows:
1600 = 200 mg/L
1800 = 100 mg/L
2000 = 50 mg/L
2200 = 25 mg/L

2. a. He has nausea and vomiting and cannot take medications by mouth. His medications will need to be given parenterally.

   b. Because of his decreased serum albumin level, a lesser amount of drugs that are usually protein bound will be bound to protein, and as a result, more free drug will be circulating and the duration of drug action may be increased. In addition, the patient has heart failure that may result in decreased cardiac output and thus decreased distribution.

   c. The patient has liver failure that will result in decreased metabolism of drugs.

   d. Because the patient's liver may not be able to effectively metabolize drugs and convert them to water-soluble compounds, excretion through the kidneys may be decreased.

3. This situation illustrates prophylactic therapy to prevent illness or other undesirable outcomes. Prophylactic intravenous antibiotic therapy may be used to prevent infection during a high-risk surgery or procedure, such as the placement of a peripherally inserted central catheter.

4. Therapeutic index is the ratio between the toxic and therapeutic concentrations of a drug. A low therapeutic index means that the range between a therapeutically active dose and a toxic dose is small. As a result, the drug has a greater likelihood of causing an adverse reaction. The nurse should monitor the patient's response carefully when a drug has a narrow therapeutic index.

CHAPTER 3
Considerations for Special Populations

Chapter Review/Critical Thinking and Application

1. c
2. a
3. d
4. b
5. b, c, d
6. d
7. b
8. e
9. a
10. c
11. It is important to keep in mind that older adults take a greater proportion of both prescription

and over-the-counter (OTC) medications and they commonly take multiple medications on a daily basis. In addition, older adults have more chronic illnesses than younger individuals. They may see several different specialists, each of whom may prescribe a set of medications. In addition, some patients self-administer OTC products to ease the discomfort of even more ailments. This use of multiple medications is termed *polypharmacy*.

12. Drawing on the information in Table 3-3 (p. 50 in the textbook), students may describe a variety of physiological changes affecting the cardiovascular, gastrointestinal, hepatic, and renal systems.

Case Study

1. Children and teenagers should not take acetylsalicytic acid (Aspirin) to treat chickenpox or influenza-like symptoms because Reye's syndrome, a rare but serious illness, has been associated with Aspirin use at these ages. It is important to check for precautions when giving any medication to children.

2. If the toddler does not like or cannot take pills, have the parent ask the pharmacist for a liquid form of the medication, which may be flavoured and better accepted than a pill.

3. The most common dosage calculation for children is the milligrams per kilogram formula. However, for over-the-counter medications, the manufacturer will convert kilograms to pounds in order to make dosing by the parents an easier process.

4. The 5-year-old child received 240 mg (at 160 mg/teaspoon, 1.5 teaspoons = 240 mg).

5. The parents should monitor the children's fever; the expected response is that the fever will go down. In addition, because the medication also has analgesic effects, signs of discomfort may decrease. The parents should also monitor for any adverse effects of the medication or worsening of the child's illness.

CHAPTER 4
Ethnocultural, Legal, and Ethical Considerations

Chapter Review/Critical Thinking and Application

1. b
2. a
3. d
4. a, b, d
5. b
6. d
7. d
8. a

9. c
10. b
11. c
12. a
13. d
14. b
15. Answers will vary depending on the group identified.
   a. Barriers may include language, poverty, access, pride, and beliefs regarding medical practices.
   b. Attitudes will vary depending on the groups identified.
   c. Questions may include the following topics: health beliefs and practices, past use of medicine, folk remedies, home remedies, use of nonprescription drugs, over-the-counter treatments, usual responses to illness, responsiveness to medical treatments, religious practices and beliefs, and dietary habits.

Case Study

1. The nurse should not give the drugs until it is established that the study has been reviewed by an institutional review board and that the patient has given informed consent. As a professional, the nurse has the responsibility to provide safe nursing care, and it is within the nurse's realm of practice to provide information and assist the patient in facing decisions regarding health care. The nurse also has the right to refuse to participate in any treatment or aspect of a patient's care that violates personal ethical principles.

2. Principles include the following:
   • Autonomy—the patient's right to self-determination. The nurse supports this by ensuring informed consent.
   • Beneficence—the doing of good. Will the patient be best served by this course of action?
   • Nonmaleficence—the duty to do no harm.
   • Veracity—the duty to tell the truth, especially with regard to investigational new drugs and informed consent.

3. Some patients believe strongly in using home remedies rather than medications. The nurse should assess and consider health beliefs and practices at the beginning of the therapeutic relationship.

4. The issue of confidentiality should be discussed. The researchers have a duty to respect privileged information about a patient. Measures that the researchers will use to ensure the confidentiality of participants should be discussed.

CHAPTER 5
Medication Errors

Chapter Review/Critical Thinking and Application

1. Medication error
2. Idiosyncratic
3. Adverse effect
4. Adverse drug reaction (ADR)
5. Adverse drug event (ADE)
6. True
7. False
8. To avoid medication errors: Follow the 10 rights of medication administration. Carefully read all drug labels and confirm that the drug, dose, time and frequency of administration, patient, and route of administration are correct. Verbal orders should be minimized but if a verbal order must be taken, repeat the order to confirm it with the prescriber, and spell the drug name aloud, speaking slowly and clearly. Never assume a route of administration; if an order is unclear or incomplete, clarify the order with the prescriber. Always read the label three times, and check the medication order before administering the medication. See the text for other possible answers.
9. Refer to Box 5-1 (p. 75 in the textbook). Chemotherapeutic drugs; neuromuscular blocking drugs; adrenergic agonists, adrenergic antagonists; opiates; thrombolytics; local anaesthetics in large containers.
10. digoxin 125 micrograms PO now
furosemide 40 mg IV daily
Discontinue all meds
NPH insulin 12 units subcutaneously with breakfast daily
garamycin otic drops, 1 drop right ear bid

Case Study

1. The nursing student should immediately inform her instructor of the error. Then together they should monitor the patient's response and follow the institution's procedure for reporting a medication error. Reporting medication errors is a professional and ethical responsibility.
2. By checking the rights of medication administration before giving this medication. In this situation, the student missed the right dose. In addition, if the student had understood the rationale for the medication (i.e., the low dose needed for antiplatelet therapy), then she might have avoided this error. One must be knowledgeable about medications and the rationale for their use in a particular patient before administering them.
3. According to Chapter 5, the recommendation is that the patient be told of the error, both as ethical practice and because of the legal implications.
4. Yes. A medication error is defined as any "preventable adverse drug event involving inappropriate medication use by a patient or health care provider"; it may or may not cause harm to the patient.
5. The Canadian Medication Incident Reporting and Prevention System (CMIRPS) exists to gather and disseminate safety information regarding medications. By reporting this error, CMIRPS is able to add to the database of medication errors and their causes and thus help identify to all health care providers the potential errors. This service is confidential.

CHAPTER 6
Patient Education and Drug Therapy

Critical Thinking and Application

1. Students should refer to the information in Chapter 25 for specific information about antihypertensive drug therapy. In addition, Table 6-1 (p. 89 in the textbook) provides information relevant to the development of teaching strategies for the 78-year-old patient.
2. Refer to Box 6-2 (p. 90 in the textbook). Ideally, a health care provider who speaks the mother's language should do the teaching. Some strategies include using pictures and illustrations, demonstrating by example, and finding an interpreter. In addition, the patient should be provided with detailed written instructions in her native language.
3. a. Answers will vary, but this nursing diagnosis should address deficient knowledge.
   b. Answers will vary, but this nursing diagnosis should address nonadherence.
4. Answers will vary, depending on the type of medication. Refer to the appropriate chapters for specific patient and family teaching and possible goals and expected outcomes.
5. Teaching plans will vary somewhat in format, but each should contain the following information:
   a. Some of the assessment items listed in the text in the section Assessment of Learning Needs Related to Drug Therapy
   b. Deficient knowledge
   c. A measurable goal with outcome criteria related to the nursing diagnosis
   d. Specific educational strategies for providing the information needed
   e. Specific questions designed to validate whether learning has occurred

Case Study

1. Both "deficient knowledge" and "nonadherence" are possible answers. In this case, "deficient knowledge" is probably the most correct because this nursing diagnosis exists when the patient has a lack of or limited understanding about his medications. For example, the pump container must be primed prior to first use. Pump the spray in the air and away from the face before using it for the first time or if it has not been used in several weeks. Spray once onto or under the tongue. In addition, he was not aware that it is important not to miss doses of antihypertensive medications. Nonadherence exists when the patient does not take the medication as directed or at all and the data collected indicate that the patient's condition has reoccurred or has not resolved. In this case, his blood pressure has improved from previous readings despite what he has said about taking his medications.

2. Answers may vary. A goal for the nursing diagnosis of "deficient knowledge" in this case may be the following: "The patient self-administers his prescribed medications on schedule without missing doses." Outcome criteria may include the following: "The patient is able to describe the schedule of medications that are ordered. The patient is able to state the rationale for consistent dosing of antihypertensive medications. The patient is able to describe the proper storage and administration of nitroglycerin spray. The patient is able to identify potential adverse effects of the prescribed medications and knows when to report them."

3. Again, answers may vary. Refer to Box 6-2. Suggestions include the following:

   - A teaching session regarding medication administration should be held with both the patient and his wife in attendance. If necessary, find out whether they have any children or neighbours nearby who may be able to assist with medications as needed.
   - Assist the patient with developing a daily time calendar for taking the prescribed medications.
   - Suggest the use of a daily or weekly pill container that can assist with reminding when doses are due. If necessary, a neighbour or the patient's son or daughter can visit periodically to fill this container.
   - Discuss and provide written literature on the purposes and adverse effects of each medication ordered and on other important issues regarding these medications.

4. Confirm whether learning has occurred by asking the patient and his wife questions related to the teaching session. Assess their understanding of the time calendar and the concept of using pill containers. Follow-up can be accomplished by telephone as needed, and a return visit to review medications can be scheduled. In addition, the patient must keep return appointments to the office so that the therapeutic outcomes of the drug therapy (i.e., blood pressure readings) can be measured.

CHAPTER 7
Over-the-Counter Drugs and Natural Health Products

Double Puzzle

Valerian
Garlic
Feverfew
St. John's wort
Ginkgo
Saw palmetto
Ginseng
Echinacea
Aloe
Goldenseal
Herbal therapy

Chapter Review/Critical Thinking and Application

1. a, b, d, f
2. d
3. a
4. b
5. c
6. Garlic, ginkgo, and ginseng
7. Older adults; children; patients with single or multiple acute and chronic illnesses; patients who are frail or in poor health; patients who are debilitated and nutritionally deficient; patients who are immunocompromised. In addition, those who have a history of renal, hepatic, cardiac, or vascular disorders may have problems with over-the-counter medications.
8. Contraindications to the use of herbal products include renal, liver, or cardiac disorders; platelet or clotting disorders; stroke or cerebral bleeding of any kind; hypertension; peptic ulcers; gastrointestinal bleeding; and any other type of abnormal bleeding. Specific contraindications exist for specific herbal products; see the text for more information.
9. Answers will vary.

Case Study

1. The Aspirin and garlic tablets may interfere with platelet and clotting functions. If the wine is taken with the kava or the valerian or both, central nervous system depression may occur.
2. Health Canada has issued a warning about the use of kava and possible liver toxicity. Also, tachyphylaxis may develop in patients who use echinacea for more than 8 weeks.
3. Because she is trying to conceive, she needs to consider the fact that the herbal agents have not been tested or proved safe for use in pregnancy. Also, acetylsalicytic acid (Aspirin) is contraindicated in pregnancy because of its antiplatelet effects.
4. Assuming the natural health products are all purchased from reputable sources in Canada and not through a foreign Web site, then the products are considered safe, because Health Canada regulations enforce standards of quality and safety assessment for all natural health products sold in Canada.
5. Many patients believe that if a product is "natural," then it is safe. The nurse should discuss each product with the patient and instruct the patient about possible contraindications, safe use, frequency of dosing, specifics about how to take the product, and the way to monitor for both therapeutic effects and complications or toxic effects.

CHAPTER 8
Vitamins and Minerals

Chapter Review/Critical Thinking and Application

1. c
2. g
3. b
4. h
5. e
6. k
7. i
8. d
9. j
10. a
11. l
12. f
13. a, d, e
14. b
15. d
16. d
17. By *endogenous*, the physician was referring to the endogenous synthesis of a form of vitamin D synthesized in the skin by ultraviolet irradiation. Dietary sources of vitamin D include fish oils, salmon, sardines, and herring; fortified milk, bread, and cereals; and animal livers, tuna fish, eggs, and butter.
18. a. Pernicious anemia
    b. The oral absorption of cyanocobalamin (vitamin B_{12} or extrinsic factor) requires the presence of the intrinsic factor, which is a glycoprotein secreted by the gastric parietal cells. Damage to the gastrointestinal tract may reduce the amount of intrinsic factor available.
    c. The patient education card for Ms. Nowaczinski should focus on foods containing cyanocobalamin; these include foods of animal origin such as liver, kidney, fish, shellfish, meat, and dairy foods.
19. To avoid venous irritation, calcium should be given via an intravenous infusion pump when given intravenously. It should be given slowly (less than 1 mL/min for adults) to avoid cardiac dysrhythmias and cardiac arrest. The physician is correct in ordering infusion with 1% procaine. This will reduce vasospasm and dilute the effects of calcium on surrounding tissues. In either case, monitor for extravasation; if it occurs, the nurse should discontinue administration immediately. The nurse should also watch for signs of hypercalcemia.
20. The orange juice contains ascorbic acid (vitamin C), which enhances the absorption of iron.

Case Study

1. The broad-spectrum antibiotics can inhibit the intestinal flora that provide the body with vitamin K_2. Consequently, a deficiency may occur. Vitamin K can be taken either orally or by injection in adults.
2. Vitamin K is essential for the synthesis of blood coagulation factors that takes place in the liver.
3. Deficiency states can also be seen in newborns because of malabsorption attributable to inadequate amounts of bile. The deficiency may also be seen in patients receiving specific anticoagulants that inhibit hepatic vitamin K activity.
4. Dietary sources of vitamin K are green leafy vegetables (cabbage, spinach, etc.), meats, and milk.

CHAPTER 9
Problematic Substance Use

Chapter Review/Critical Thinking and Application

1. h
2. i
3. f

4. e
5. g
6. d
7. j
8. a
9. c
10. b
11. c
12. d
13. b, c, e
14. c
15. b
16. The nicotine transdermal system (patch) and nicotine polacrilex (gum) can be used to provide nicotine without the carcinogens in tobacco. The patches provide a stepwise reduction in delivery and work by gradually reducing the nicotine dose over time. With use of the gum, rapid chewing releases an immediate dose of nicotine, but this dose is approximately one half of what the average smoker receives from one cigarette, and the onset of action is longer than with smoking. Therefore, the reinforcement and self-reward effects of smoking are minimized. Zyban is a sustained-release form of the antidepressant bupropion and is the first nicotine-free prescription medicine used to treat nicotine dependence.
17. For all three levels of ethanol withdrawal, benzodiazepines such as diazepam (Valium, Vivol), lorazepam (Ativan), and chlordiazepoxide (Librax) are used in various doses and frequencies. The doses are lower for "mild" withdrawal; for "moderate" ethanol withdrawal, higher doses of the benzodiazepines are used and dosage is tapered over 5 days as needed. For "severe" withdrawal, also known as *delirium tremens*, the dosages of diazepam, lorazepam, or chlordiazepine are at their highest until the patient's agitation has subsided. In addition, thiamine injections may be given.

Case Study

1. Ethanol causes central nervous system depression.
2. Acute severe alcoholic intoxication may cause cardiovascular depression and long-term excessive use has largely irreversible effects on the heart. Moderate amounts may either stimulate or depress respirations, but large amounts produce lethal respiratory depression.
3. First, the nurse should monitor the patient's respiratory and cardiovascular status and prevent injury from falling or aspiration from vomiting. In addition, the nurse should be alert to the patient's behaviour and mental status to identify changes in his condition. Withdrawal from alcohol can lead to serious conditions such as delirium tremens (see question 4). Careful assessment of vital signs and mental status is imperative at this time; early withdrawal symptoms may be an increase in blood pressure and pulse with an altered mental status.
4. Mr. Chan should stay in the hospital for observation and possible treatment of delirium tremens, which may begin with tremors and agitation and progress to hallucinations and sometimes death. See Box 9-6 (p. 141 in the textbook) for information on treatment of ethanol withdrawal.
5. Chronic excessive ingestion of ethanol is directly associated with several serious mental and neurological disorders. Nutritional and vitamin B deficiencies can occur that result in conditions such as Wernicke's encephalopathy, Korsakoff's psychosis, polyneuritis, and nicotinic acid deficiency encephalopathy. Seizures may also occur. In addition, long-term ingestion of ethanol may result in alcoholic hepatitis or liver cirrhosis.

CHAPTER 10
Photo Atlas of Drug Administration

Chapter Review/Critical Thinking and Application

1. b
2. c
3. a
4. b
5. c
6. c
7. b
8. a
9. c
10. a
11. b
12. d
13. b
14. a
15. a, b, c, e
16. a. Palpate sites for masses or tenderness and assess the amount of subcutaneous tissue.
    b. Note the integrity and size of the muscle and palpate for tenderness.
    c. Note any lesions or discolouration of the forearm.
17. See descriptions under Injections Overview in the textbook for each type of injection.
18. Remove the needle, and ensure that the site is not bleeding. Discard the medication and syringe, draw up new medication, and repeat the procedure in a different location.

19. Rather than pouring it into a medication cup, draw small volumes of liquid medications into a calibrated oral syringe.
20. 250 divided by 4 (4 puffs/day) would equal 62.5 days.

Case Study

1. For the adult, the ventrogluteal site is the preferred injection site. If the woman is of average size, choose a needle that is 4 cm long and 21 to 25 gauge and insert the needle at a 90-degree angle. For an infant, the preferred site is the vastus lateralis site. The needle should be of the correct length to ensure that it reaches muscle tissue, not the subcutaneous layer.
2. For an infant or child younger than 3 years of age, the pinna of the ear should be pulled down and back before the drops are administered. The drops should be directed along the sides of the ear rather than directly onto the eardrum. The drops should be taken out of refrigeration about 30 minutes before giving them. The mother should stay with her child and ensure that she lies on her side for 5 to 10 minutes. Gentle massage of the tragus area of the ear with her finger will help distribute the medication down the ear canal.
3. Liquid medication doses under 5 mL should be drawn up in a calibrated oral syringe.
4. Liquids are usually ordered because infants cannot swallow pills or capsules. A plastic disposable oral dosing syringe is recommended for measuring small doses of liquid medications. Position the infant so that the head is slightly elevated. Place the plastic dropper or syringe inside the infant's mouth, beside the tongue, and administer the liquid in small amounts while allowing the infant to swallow each time. Take great care to prevent aspiration. A crying infant can easily aspirate medication. Do not add the medication to a bottle of formula. The infant may refuse the feeding or may not drink all of it and, as a result, would not receive the entire dosage of medication.

CHAPTER 11
Analgesic Drugs

Critical Thinking Crossword

Across
2. Agonist
6. Superficial
7. Pain tolerance
10. Threshold
12. Opioid

13. Partial
14. Abstinence

Down
1. Antagonist
3. Chronic
4. Visceral
5. Opiate
6. Somatic
8. Acute
9. Compulsive
11. Adjuvant

Chapter Review

1. b
2. d
3. c
4. d
5. b, c, e
6. g
7. f
8. i
9. h
10. d
11. b
12. j
13. c
14. a
15. e

Case Study

1. Superficial pain, which originates from the skin or mucous membranes
2. A back rub. Massage to the affected area often decreases the pain. When an area is rubbed or liniment is applied to an area, large sensory fibres from peripheral receptors carry impulses to the spinal cord. This causes impulse transmission to be inhibited and the gate to be closed. This in turn reduces the recognition of the pain impulses arriving by means of the small fibres. This is the same pathway that the opioid analgesics use to alleviate pain.
3. All opioids cause some histamine release. It is thought that this histamine release is responsible for many of the unwanted adverse effects, such as itching.
4. The most serious adverse effect of opioids is central nervous depression, which may lead to respiratory depression. Naloxone, an opioid reversal agent, may need to be administered to reverse severe respiratory depression.
5. The use of a nonopioid analgesic with an opioid is known as *adjuvant analgesic therapy*. This allows the use of smaller doses of opioids,

which accomplishes two important functions. First, it diminishes some of the adverse effects that are seen with higher doses of opioids, such as respiratory depression, constipation, and urinary retention. Second, adjuvant therapy approaches the pain stimulus from another mechanism and has a resulting synergistic beneficial effect in reducing the pain.

CHAPTER 12
General and Local Anaesthetics

Critical Thinking Crossword

Across

3. Pancuronium
6. General
7. Topical
8. Adjunctive
9. Local

Down

1. Atropine
2. Anaesthetics
3. Parenteral
4. Balanced
5. Regional

Chapter Review/Critical Thinking and Application

1. a, c, e
2. b
3. a
4. b
5. b, c, e
6. c
7. 1 = c; 2 = a; 3 = b
8. Children are more susceptible to problems such as central nervous depression, toxicity, atelectasis, pneumonia, and cardiac abnormalities because their hepatic, cardiac, respiratory, and renal systems are not fully developed or fully functional.
9. These agents cause paralysis but not anaesthesia. The patient is still able to hear the nurse and feel touch. It is important to remain professional at all times and to take the time to orient the patient to his surroundings, to what noises mean, and to what the nurse is going to be doing to him.
10. Mrs. Edwards will be given a combination of intravenous medications that will produce analgesia and also amnesia of the procedure, but she will still be alert enough to breathe on her own and follow verbal directions as needed. In some cases, local anaesthesia will be used to enhance patient comfort. This type of sedation is called *moderate sedation*; it is associated with

fewer complications than general anaesthesia and a shorter recovery time.

Case Study

1. In balanced anaesthesia, minimal doses of a combination of anaesthetic drugs (both intravenous and inhaled) are used to achieve the desired level of anaesthesia for the surgical procedure. Adjunctive drugs may also be used and commonly include sedative–hypnotics, narcotics, and neuromuscular blocking agents (NMBAs) (depolarizing drugs such as succinylcholine and the nondepolarizing or competitive drugs such as atracurium [Nimbex] and pancuronium). Combining several different drugs makes it possible for general anaesthesia to be accomplished with smaller amounts of anaesthetic gases and thus reduces the adverse effects.
2. The main therapeutic use of the NMBA succinylcholine is to maintain controlled ventilation during surgical procedures. When respiratory muscles are paralyzed by NMBAs, mechanical ventilation is easier because the body's drive to control respirations is eliminated by the drug; this allows the ventilator to have total control of the respirations.
3. Multiple medical conditions (listed in Box 12-4 on p. 227 of the textbook) can predispose an individual to toxicity. These conditions increase the sensitivity of an individual to NMBAs and prolong their effects. Because the patient's temperature has decreased, hypothermia may lead to an increased sensitivity to the medication.
4. Anticholinesterase drugs such as neostigmine are antidotes and are used to reverse the muscle paralysis.
5. Local anaesthesia is most commonly used in settings in which loss of consciousness, whole-body relaxation, and loss of unresponsiveness are either unnecessary or not wanted. A lower incidence of toxic effects is associated with the use of local anaesthetics because little is systemically absorbed.
6. Regardless of the type of anaesthesia a patient is receiving, one of the most important nursing considerations during this time is close and frequent observation of the patient and all body systems, with specific attention to the ABCs of nursing care (*a*irway, *b*reathing, and *c*irculation) and vital signs. Resuscitative equipment, as well as any antidote, should be kept nearby in case of cardiorespiratory distress or arrest, as well as any drug antidote. Other nursing actions include monitoring

all aspects of body functions (including the ABCs of care), instituting safety measures, and implementing the physician's orders.

CHAPTER 13
Central Nervous System Depressants and Muscle Relaxants

Chapter Review/Critical Thinking and Application

1. a
2. b
3. a
4. d
5. c
6. d
7. Answers should reflect the discussion under Toxicity and Management of Overdose in the textbook. The priority of care would be to maintain the ABCs (*a*irway, *b*reathing, *c*irculation), particularly respirations, because respiratory depression is likely.
8. Benzodiazepines can be used for insomnia only if they are limited to short-term use (less than 2 to 4 weeks). With long-term use, rebound insomnia and severe withdrawal can develop. If Jackie needs to take something to help her sleep while she is on her trip, the nonbenzodiazepine hypnotics may be an option; and, of course, the nurse can provide patient teaching on nonpharmacological methods to aid sleep.
9. Older adults should be started on lower doses because they generally experience a more pronounced effect from benzodiazepines.
10. a. Ask about allergies, central nervous system disorders, sleep disorders, diabetes, addictive disorders, personality disorders, thyroid conditions, and kidney and liver function status.
    b. Other measures should include alcohol and central nervous system depressants, but also all prescribed or over-the-counter medications.
    c. The patient's age matters because these drugs have increased effects in older adults and small children.
11. a. Patient teaching should include information about potential adverse effects and potential drug interactions. In addition, safety measures to prevent injury stemming from decreased sensorium must be emphasized.
    b. These medications are most effective when used in conjunction with rest and physical therapy.
12. *Tachyphylaxis* is the rapid appearance of a progressive decrease in response to a pharmacologically or physiologically active substance after its repetitive administration.

Chloral hydrate, an older nonbarbiturate sedative–hypnotic drug, has this characteristic. This occurrence of tachyphylaxis is a disadvantage because tachyphylaxis makes the drug useful only for short-term therapy.

Case Study

1. Barbiturates are considered controlled substances because of the potential for misuse and the severe effects that result if they are not used appropriately. Other hypnotic drugs are now used more frequently than barbiturates because they have fewer adverse effects and are safer than the older barbiturates. They also do not suppress rapid eye movement (REM) sleep to the same extent as do barbiturates.
2. Barbiturates deprive people of REM sleep (dreaming sleep), and long-term use can result in agitation and inability to deal with normal stress. In addition, when the barbiturate is stopped, the returning REM sleep may be more intense than before and lead to nightmares (a rebound effect). Barbiturates are habit forming, they have a low therapeutic index, and severe withdrawal effects may occur when the medication is stopped. Other drugs have been shown to be safer to use for treatment of insomnia.
3. Other central nervous system depressants, particularly alcohol, should be avoided. There may also be an additive effect with the intake of the natural health product valerian.
4. Zopiclone (Imovane) is indicated for the short-term treatment of insomnia and has been shown to be effective for up to 5 weeks. Zopiclone has a short half-life, thus the patient should be taught that if sleep difficulties include early awakenings, a dose can be taken as long as it is at least 4 hours before the patient must arise. In addition, the patient should explore other nonpharmacological options to use for the treatment of insomnia and try to find the cause of the sleep problems. See Box 13-1 (p. 253 in the textbook) for information on nonpharmacological measures to promote sleep.

CHAPTER 14
Antiepileptic Drugs

Critical Thinking Crossword

Across
2. Emergency
6. Primary
10. Hepatotoxicity
11. Seizure
12. Slowly

Down
1. Secondary
3. Convulsion
4. Benzodiazepines
5. Idiopathic
6. Phenobarbital
7. Autoinduction
8. Epilepsy
9. Phenytoin

Chapter Review/Critical Thinking and Application

1. d
2. a
3. b, c, d
4. c
5. b
6. c
7. Carbamazepine undergoes autoinduction, the process by which the metabolism of a drug increases over time, which leads to lower-than-expected drug concentrations.
8. Jeremy's mother should be told that topiramate should be taken whole and should not be crushed, broken in half, or chewed. It does have a bitter taste and seems to be better tolerated when taken with food. She can still give it with gelatin, as long as the dosage form remains whole.

Case Study

1. Generalized seizures, more specifically, absence seizures. These are most common in children.
2. The succinimide ethosuximide (Zarontin) is indicated for treatment of absence seizures in children. See Table 14-1 on p. 259 of the textbook.
3. Mattie's mother needs to be sure to measure the dose carefully with an exact graduated device or oral syringe, rather than with a household teaspoon, and to give the medication at the same time daily. She should report excessive sedation, confusion, lethargy, or decreased movement. See Patient Education (p. 268 of the textbook) for more information.
4. Mattie's mother should be encouraged to keep a journal to record Mattie's signs and symptoms before, during, and after any seizure activity in order to measure the therapeutic effectiveness of the medication.
5. A therapeutic response to antiepileptic drugs does not mean the patient has been cured of the seizures but that seizure activity is decreased or absent. Further evaluation will be needed before a decision is made to stop the medication. Treatment may need to last for years or may be lifelong.

CHAPTER 15
Antiparkinsonian Drugs

Chapter Review/Critical Thinking and Application

1. b
2. a
3. c
4. c
5. a, c
6. d
7. a. Dopamine must be given in this form because exogenously administered dopamine cannot pass through the blood–brain barrier; levodopa can.
   b. The addition of carbidopa avoids the high peripheral levels of dopamine and the unwanted adverse effects induced by the large doses of levodopa necessary when the drug is given alone.
   c. Carbidopa does not cross the blood–brain barrier and thus prevents levodopa breakdown in the periphery. This in turn allows levodopa to reach and cross the blood–brain barrier without carbidopa doing so. Once in the brain, the levodopa is then broken down to dopamine, which can be used directly.
8. The nurse must ask whether Mrs. Chatterjee is lactating; if so, amantadine is contraindicated.
9. Older adults, particularly men who have a diagnosis of benign prostatic hypertrophy, are at risk for urinary retention. Jane's neighbour may or may not have that condition, but his age is a major factor. Jane's age is not a concern at this time. This drug may also cause palpitations.

Case Study

1. The primary cause of Parkinson's disease is an imbalance in the two neurotransmitters dopamine and acetylcholine (ACh) in the basal ganglia of the brain. This imbalance is caused by a failure of the nerve terminals in the substantia nigra to produce dopamine, which acts in the basal ganglia to control body movements. A correct balance between dopamine and ACh is needed for the proper regulation of posture, muscle tone, and voluntary movement. The deficiency of dopamine can also lead to excessive ACh activity due to the lack of dopamine's normal balancing effect. Symptoms of Parkinson's disease do not appear until approximately 80% of the dopamine store in the substantia nigra of the basal ganglia has been depleted.
2. Drug therapy is aimed at increasing the levels of dopamine at the remaining functioning

nerve terminals. It is also aimed at blocking the effects of ACh and slowing the progression of the disease.

3. Amantadine facilitates the release of dopamine from nerve endings that are still intact. The result is higher levels of dopamine in the central nervous system.

4. Amantadine is most effective in the early stages of Parkinson's disease, but as the disease progresses and the number of functioning nerves diminishes, amantadine's effect is also reduced. It is usually effective for only 6 to 12 months.

5. The patient with Parkinson's disease often experiences rapid swings in response to levodopa; this fluctuating response is known as the *on-off phenomenon*. This phenomenon is seen in patients taking levodopa for a long time. Such patients may experience periods when they have good control ("on" time) and periods when they have bad control or breakthrough Parkinson's disease ("off" time). Carbidopa is a peripheral decarboxylase inhibitor that does not cross the blood–brain barrier. As a result, carbidopa prevents levodopa from breaking down in the periphery and allows more levodopa to reach and cross the blood–brain barrier. Levodopa–carbidopa combinations, such as Sinemet CR, may help reduce the "off" periods.

CHAPTER 16

Psychotherapeutic Drugs

Chapter Review/Critical Thinking and Application

1. c
2. b
3. c
4. a, c, d
5. d
6. m
7. g
8. h
9. o
10. b
11. j
12. k
13. l
14. c
15. n
16. a
17. d
18. i
19. f
20. e

21. a. If Viktor is taking a benzodiazepine for anxiety and drinking alcohol, he is probably experiencing benzodiazepine toxicity or overdose.
   b. If ingestion is recent (within 4 hours), Viktor might be treated with activated charcoal, and a cathartic may be administered. He might be given flumazenil (Anexate) to reverse the effect of a more severe benzodiazepine overdose.

22. a. Mr. Delvecchio needs to be aware of the foods and drinks, including red wine, that he can no longer have because they contain tyramine.
   b. It appears that Mr. Delvecchio may have inadvertently ingested something containing tyramine, which has caused a hypertensive crisis.

23. Second-generation antidepressants offer an advantage over other antidepressants because they have fewer and less severe adverse effects.

24. If the antidepressant taken is a first-generation antidepressant, or tricyclic, excessive dosages can result in lethal cardiac dysrhythmias as well as seizures. Dysrhythmias are responsible for most deaths due to overdoses.

Case Study

1. See Table 16-3 (p. 293 of the textbook) for potential adverse effects for benzodiazepines. Most are related to the effects on the central nervous system. Patient teaching includes warning the patient to avoid driving or operating heavy equipment or machinery until he becomes accustomed to the adverse effects of the medication. In addition, measures should be taken to avoid orthostatic hypotension. Finally, he should avoid alcohol and other central nervous depressants while taking this medication.

2. If Gene is experiencing life-altering anxiety, then he should also consider undergoing psychotherapy to assist him at this time.

3. Benzodiazepines are potentially habit forming and addictive, with possible withdrawal symptoms such as anxiety, panic attacks, convulsions, nausea, and vomiting. The medication should not be withdrawn abruptly. Patients should always be advised to take the medication as directed and never to stop taking the medication abruptly.

4. There is a potential for benzodiazepines to cause serious life-threatening toxicities, but when taken alone in normal doses in otherwise healthy patients, they are safe and effective anxiolytics. When taken with other sedating

medications or with alcohol, however, life-threatening respiratory depression or arrest can occur. An overdose of benzodiazepines may result in one or more of the following symptoms: somnolence, confusion, coma, and respiratory depression. Overdose may be treated with administration of activated charcoal and a cathartic. The benzodiazepine-specific antidote flumazenil (Anexate) may be used in severe cases.

5. Buspirone has the advantages of being both nonsedating and non–habit forming compared with benzodiazepines.

CHAPTER 17
Central Nervous System Stimulant Drugs

Chapter Review/Critical Thinking and Application

1. b
2. b, c, e
3. a
4. c
5. d
6. b
7. a. Stacey has narcolepsy.
    b. Methylphenidate, an amphetamine, may be ordered.
    c. Amphetamines increase mental alertness, increase motor activity, and diminish the patient's sense of fatigue by stimulating the cerebral cortex and possibly the reticular activating system.
    d. (i) Stacey should take her medication exactly as her physician prescribes, without skipping, omitting, or doubling up on the doses.
       (ii) Stacey should avoid other sources of central nervous system stimulants, particularly caffeine-containing products (e.g., coffee, tea, colas, and chocolate). She should check with her doctor before taking any over-the-counter drug, and she should not consume any substance that contains alcohol.
8. Weight loss due to anorexia is associated with drugs used for the management of attention deficit hyperactivity disorder, and so it is important to monitor for weight gain or loss in children who are taking these drugs. Height and weight should be measured and recorded before therapy is initiated and growth rate should be plotted during therapy. Nutritional status should be assessed with attention to daily dietary intake as well as the amount eaten before drug therapy and after therapy is initiated.
9. With orlistat (Xenical), patients need to watch dietary fat intake. Restricting the intake of fat to less than 30% of total caloric intake may help in decreasing the occurrence of the gastrointestinal adverse effects. In addition, orlistat is to be taken with meals that contain fat. Supplementation with fat-soluble vitamins may be indicated.
10. These drugs work to reduce the severity of the headaches but do not prevent headaches.

Case Study

1. Serotonin agonists work by stimulating 5-HT$_1$ receptors in the brain. This stimulation results in constriction of dilated blood vessels in the brain and decreased release of inflammatory neuropeptides.
2. Orally administered medications often may not be tolerated because of the nausea and vomiting that often accompany the headaches. Alternative formulations such as subcutaneous self-injections and nasal sprays are advantageous. They also have a more rapid onset of action, producing relief in some patients in 10 to 15 minutes compared with 1 to 2 hours with tablets.
3. The use of sumatriptan succinate (Imitrex DF) is contraindicated in patients with ischemic heart disease, signs and symptoms consistent with ischemic heart disease, Prinzmetal's angina, and uncontrolled hypertension.
4. Foods containing tyramine should be avoided because tyramine is known to precipitate severe headaches. Tyramine-containing foods include beer, wine, aged cheese, food additives, preservatives, artificial sweeteners, chocolate, and caffeine.
5. Keeping a journal of the occurrence of headaches, precipitating factors, and response to drug therapy is also encouraged in order to follow the patient's progress and response to drug therapy.

CHAPTER 18
Adrenergic Drugs

Chapter Review/Critical Thinking and Application

1. d
2. b, d
3. a, b, d
4. a
5. c
6. The α-adrenergic activity of this drug causes vasoconstriction in the nasal mucosa. This produces shrinkage of the mucosa and promotes easier nasal breathing.
7. Use of the drug is contraindicated in patients who have a tumour that secretes catecholamines, such as a pheochromocytoma.

8. The action of dopamine depends on the dose. At low doses, dopamine can dilate blood vessels in the brain, heart, kidneys, and mesentery, increasing blood flow to these areas. Increased renal blood flow may help remove excess fluid volume. At higher infusion rates, dopamine can improve contractility and cardiac output.

9. The toxic effects of adrenergic drugs are mainly an extension of their common adverse effects, such as seizures, hypotension or hypertension, dysrhythmias, and other effects, but the two most life-threatening toxic effects involve the central nervous system and cardiovascular system. Seizures can be effectively managed with diazepam. An extreme elevation in blood pressure poses the risk of hemorrhage in the brain and elsewhere in the body. To lower the blood pressure quickly, a rapid-acting α-adrenergic–blocking drug can be used to reverse the adrenergic effects. Most of the adrenergic drugs have short half-lives, and therefore their effects are relatively short-lived. Stopping the drug should quickly cause the toxic symptoms to subside. The treatment of overdoses often involves treating the symptoms and supporting the patient's respiratory and cardiac functions.

10. a. Derk is probably having an anaphylactic reaction to the antbiotic.
    b. The nurse's first response should be to stop the medication. The nurse then should notify the physician and stay with the patient to monitor and support the ABCs (*a*irway, *b*reathing, and *c*irculation).
    c. Epinephrine is the drug of choice for anaphylactic reactions.

Case Study

1. Before giving this medication, the nurse should assess for hypersensitivity to salbutamol and assess breath sounds and vital signs (blood pressure, pulse rate, respiratory rate) to obtain a baseline for comparative purposes. Because this medication may cause tachycardia and cardiac dysrhythmias, Maureen's pulse rate and rhythm should be monitored during the treatment. Afterward, Maureen's vital signs and breath sounds should be assessed again, as well as her therapeutic response to the medication.

2. Salbutamol given orally has an onset of action of 30 minutes and peaks in 2.5 hours. Inhaled salbutamol has an onset of action of 5 to 15 minutes and peaks in 1 to 1.5 hours. Therefore, the inhaled form will take effect faster than the oral form.

3. These are expected adverse effects of the salbutamol and will soon wear off.

4. Salmeterol is indicated for asthma and the prevention of bronchospasms in patients who may need long-term maintenance of their asthma. Patients should be taught that salmeterol is not to be used for relief of acute symptoms, and education about its dosing is important. Dosing of salmeterol is usually at two puffs twice daily 12 hours apart for maintenance. For prevention of exercise-induced asthma, the recommendation is two puffs 30 minutes to 1 hour before exercise and no additional dosing for 12 hours. If Maureen is still taking the inhaled steroid, then the bronchodilator should be taken first, and then she should wait approximately 5 minutes before taking the steroid inhaler. All equipment should be rinsed, and the patient should be encouraged to perform mouth care after the use of any inhaled forms of medication.

CHAPTER 19
Adrenergic-Blocking Drugs

Chapter Review/Critical Thinking and Application

1. a, b, d
2. a
3. c
4. b
5. d
6. Extravasation can cause vasoconstriction and ultimately tissue death (necrosis). If the vasoconstriction is not reversed quickly, the whole limb can be lost. Phentolamine, an α-blocker, can reverse this potent vasoconstriction and restore blood flow to the ischemic, vasoconstricted area. When phentolamine is injected subcutaneously in a circular fashion around the extravasation site, it causes α-adrenergic receptor blockade and vasodilation. This in turn increases blood flow to the ischemic tissue, thus preventing permanent damage.

7. Some ß-blockers are considered cardioprotective because they inhibit stimulation by the circulating catecholamines released during muscle damage, such as that caused by a myocardial infarction. When a ß-blocker occupies their receptors, the circulating catecholamines cannot bind to their receptors. Thus the ß-blockers protect the heart from being stimulated by these catecholamines, which would only further increase the heart rate and the contractile force, thereby increasing myocardial oxygen demand.

8. Ms. Clarkson should take her apical pulse for 1 full minute and monitor her blood pressure because cardiac depression can occur with these drugs. If her systolic blood pressure decreases to less than 100 mmHg or her pulse decreases to less than 60 beats/min, she should contact her physician. She should also report any weight gain, especially of more than 1 kg in 24 hours or 2 kg in a week, as well as any weakness, shortness of breath, or edema.

9. A common problem with the α_1-blockers such as prazosin is that when pateints first start taking these drugs, they may experience lightheadedness and orthostatic hypotension. Patients should quickly develop a tolerance to this effect. Mr. Sniders should be taught to take care when standing up to prevent falling if he gets lightheaded; taking the first dose at bedtime may help.

Case Study

1. Nonselective ß-blockers (which block both $ß_1$ and $ß_2$ receptors) may precipitate bradycardia and hypotension; their use is contraindicated in asthma. Therefore, if the patient has heart disease as well as respiratory disease, then a $ß_1$-blocker, or "cardioselective" drug, would be beneficial because it would not produce constriction or increased airway resistance as would $ß_2$-blockers.

2. When a ß-blocker is given, it occupies receptors and prevents circulating catecholamines (which are released when a myocardial infarction occurs) from binding to these receptors. The ß-blocker thus prevents stimulation of the heart by these catecholamines, which would only further increase heart rate, contractile force, and myocardial oxygen demand. In addition, cardioselective $ß_1$-blockers such as atenolol block the $ß_1$-adrenergic receptors on the surface of the heart. This reduces myocardial stimulation, which in turn reduces heart rate, slows conduction through the atrioventricular node, prolongs sinoatrial node recovery, and decreases myocardial oxygen demand by decreasing myocardial contractile force (contractility).

3. Table 19-3 (p. 368 in the textbook) lists ß-blocker–induced adverse effects. Patient teaching should include instructions to monitor the apical pulse for 1 full minute and monitor blood pressure because of the cardiac depression that can occur, and to notify the physician if systolic blood pressure decreases to lower than 100 mmHg or pulse decreases to less than 60 beats/min. Patients should also report any weight gain, especially a gain of 1 kg or more in a 24-hour period or 2 kg or more in a week, as well as any weakness, shortness of breath, and edema. The patient should also be taught about orthostatic changes and cautioned to rise slowly when getting up to avoid syncope. For other teaching tips, see Patient Education (p. 374 in the textbook).

4. Make sure that patients are weaned off these medications slowly, if this is indicated, because of the possible rebound hypertension or chest pain that rapid withdrawal can precipitate.

CHAPTER 20
Cholinergic Drugs

Chapter Review/Critical Thinking and Application

1. h
2. g
3. f
4. b
5. j
6. e
7. i
8. a
9. c
10. b
11. b
12. d
13. c
14. b, c, d, f
15. a
16. SLUDGE stands for *Sa*livation, *L*acrimation, *U*rinary incontinence, *D*iarrhea, *G*astrointestinal cramps, and *E*mesis.
17. a. Bethanechol is the drug of choice.
    b. None. Bethanechol is contraindicated in patients with a genitourinary obstruction. The drug should be discontinued immediately.
18. a. Cholinergic crisis
    b. Ensure that atropine, the antidote, is readily available.
19. a. Ms. Bethke should experience less eyelid drooping (ptosis), less double vision (diplopia), less difficulty swallowing and chewing, and less weakness.
    b. Ms. Bethke should report any increased muscle weakness, abdominal cramps, diarrhea, or difficulty breathing.

Case Study

1. There are no "cures" for Alzheimer's disease, but there are several drugs available for management of symptoms. Their use can sometimes yield

enough improvement in a patient's mental status to make a noticeable improvement in the quality of life for patients as well as caregivers and family members. However, individual response to these medications does vary from patient to patient. Available drugs include donepezil (Aricept), galantamine (Reminyl), rivastigmine (Exelon), and memantine (Ebixa).

2. Because of Arthur's history of hepatitis A, caution should be taken if galantamine hydrobromide (Reminyl) is chosen; the dose of this drug should be reduced for patients with moderately reduced renal or hepatic function. Results of liver function studies should be monitored if he is given this medication.

3. Direct-acting cholinergic agonists bind to cholinergic receptors and activate them. Indirect-acting cholinergic agonists act by making more acetylcholine (ACh) available at the receptor site. As a result, ACh binds to and stimulates the receptor. They do this by inhibiting cholinesterase, the enzyme responsible for breaking down ACh.

4. Adverse effects of rivastigmine include dizziness, headache, nausea and vomiting, diarrhea, and anorexia (loss of appetite). Administering this drug with meals helps decrease the gastrointestinal side effects even though absorption may be decreased, too. Patients who become dizzy with the therapy should be assisted with ambulation.

5. Memantine (Ebixa), an N-methyl-D-aspartate (NMBA) receptor antagonist, has been conditionally approved by Health Canada for the management of symptoms in patients with moderate to advanced Alzheimer's disease. Memantine exerts its therapeutic effect through its action on the NMDA receptors, thus blocking the effects of pathologically elevated and sustained levels of glutamate. It is these elevated levels of glutamate that are thought to lead to neuron dysfunction. Memantine may slow the decline of memory and cognition in Alzheimer's disease. This drug is not suitable for Arthur because he has mild Alzheimer's disease.

CHAPTER 21
Cholinergic-Blocking Drugs

Chapter Review/Critical Thinking and Application

1. a
2. a, c, d
3. b
4. c
5. b

6. Atropine sulfate is used preoperatively to reduce salivation and excessive secretions in the respiratory and gastrointestinal tracts. Glycopyrrolate is also used for this purpose.

7. a. Initially, Mr. Aziz should be treated with hospitalization and close, continuous monitoring (including continuous electrocardiographic monitoring). Consultation with a Poison Control Centre is recommended. Activated charcoal can be administered to remove drug that is already absorbed. Fluid therapy and other standard measures used to treat shock should be instituted as needed.

   b. In the case of hallucinations, physostigmine has proved helpful, although its use is somewhat controversial because of severe adverse effects with routine use; it is available in Canada only under the Special Access Programme.

8. Antihistamines can have additive effects with cholinergic blockers, resulting in increased effects.

9. a. In the treatment of symptomatic bradycardia, higher dosages of atropine result in an increase in heart rate because of the cholinergic-blocking effects on the heart's conduction system. Atropine blocks the inhibitory vagal (cholinergic) effects on the pacemaker cells of the sinoatrial and atrioventricular nodes, which can lead to an increased heart rate due to unopposed sympathetic stimulation.

   b. Atropine has a therapeutic effect in cases of exposure to organophosphate insecticides because of its anticholinesterase effects.

Case Study

1. Tolterodine (Detrol) should not be used in patients with narrow-angle glaucoma or urinary retention. Mrs. Walsh's "eye problems" should be evaluated further.

2. Tolterodine appears to cause a much lower incidence of dry mouth. This may be due to tolterodine's specificity for the bladder as opposed to the salivary glands.

3. When these cholinergic-blocking agents are used to treat urinary incontinence, the inability to sweat or perspire should be managed with an increase in fluids and avoidance of extreme heat. Mrs. Walsh needs to avoid overheating when working outside.

4. Although this drug may have a lower incidence of dry mouth, it may still cause this unpleasant adverse effect because it is a cholinergic-blocking drug. Dry mouth is managed best by drinking adequate fluids, chewing gum, performing frequent mouth care, sucking

on sugar-free hard candy, and using saliva substitute (artificial saliva) products such as Moi-Stir, available in pharmacies.

CHAPTER 22
Positive Inotropic Drugs

Chapter Review/Critical Thinking and Application

1. b
2. c
3. c
4. a
5. b
6. a, c, d, f
7. Vomiting, headache, fatigue, and dysrhythmia are adverse effects of cardiac glycosides. The presence of a serum potassium level of greater than 5 mmol/L, along with these symptoms, means that administration of digoxin immune Fab is indicated for the treatment of severe digoxin toxicity.
8. Because of digoxin's long duration of action and half-life, the physician has prescribed a loading, or "digitalizing," dose for Mr. Ali to bring the serum levels of the drug up to a therapeutic level more quickly. The usual loading dose is 1 to 1.5 mg/day, whereas the usual maintenance dose is 0.125 to 0.5 mg/day.
9. The therapeutic window is the range of drug levels in the blood that is considered therapeutic. Drug levels below this range would be subtherapeutic, and drug levels above this range may be toxic. Because digoxin has such a narrow therapeutic window, patients require constant monitoring for adverse effects and toxic symptoms.
10. Increased urinary output and decreased dyspnea and fatigue are therapeutic effects of digoxin. The constipation needs to be assessed. Mr. Ferris should not be allowed to consume large amounts of bran or other foods high in fibre because the bran will bind to the digitalis and make less of the drug available for absorption.
11. a. Milrinone lactate increases the force of contraction (inotropic effect) and relaxes the blood vessels, causing a reduction in afterload, or the force against which the heart must pump to eject its volume.
    b. Phosphodiesterase inhibitors do not stimulate receptors to cause an increase in the force of contraction as other inotropic drugs do, and therefore the drug maintains its effectiveness for a longer period of time. As a result, increased dosages are not needed to maintain positive results; thus, unwanted cardiac adverse effects do not occur.
    c. Dysrhythmia, mainly ventricular

Case Study

1. Positive inotropic effect: increases myocardial contractility
   Negative chronotropic effect: decreases the heart rate
   Negative dromotropic effect: slows the conduction of electrical impulses in the heart
2. Effects on:
   • Stroke volume: increased
   • Venous blood pressure and vein engorgement: decreased
   • Coronary circulation: increased
   • Diuresis: increased due to improved circulation
3. First, the nurse should complete an assessment by checking the patient's apical pulse, heart and lung sounds, and blood pressure. In addition, her potassium level should be checked because low levels of potassium may lead to digoxin toxicity. The patient should be monitored for signs of digoxin toxicity, particularly dangerous dysrhythmias. The digoxin level of 3.5 ng/mL is above the therapeutic range.

CHAPTER 23
Antidysrhythmic Drugs

Chapter Review/Critical Thinking and Application

1. d
2. c
3. a
4. d
5. a
6. b
7. a, (3); b, (1); c, (2)
8. a. Class II antidysrhythmics, or ß-blockers, are indicated because they have been shown to significantly reduce the incidence of sudden cardiac death after myocardial infarction.
   b. If Mr. Killian had asthma, use of most of the class II drugs would be contraindicated. Noncardioselective ß-blockers block not only the $ß_1$-adrenergic receptors in the heart but also the $ß_2$-adrenergic receptors in the lungs. As a result, preexisting asthma could be worsened.
9. Amiodarone (Cordarone) is considered a drug of last resort. Although it is effective, amiodarone can penetrate and concentrate in the adipose tissue of any organ in the body, where it may cause unwanted effects. It may cause either hypothyroidism or hyperthyroidism, corneal microdeposits, pulmonary toxicity, and even dysrhythmias.

Amiodarone has a long half-life, and the adverse effects may take months to subside.

10. a. Lidocaine must be injected intramuscularly or intravenously; when lidocaine is taken orally, the liver converts most of it to inactive metabolites.
    b. Lidocaine is extensively metabolized in the liver. For patients in liver failure or with a history of cirrhosis, as with Mr. Kowalski, a dosage reduction of 50% is recommended.

11. Mrs. Inez should *not* double up on her medication. The physician should be contacted about the missed dose and about Mrs. Inez's symptoms of chest pain and dizziness, which are adverse effects of the quinidine.

Case Study

1. As their name implies, calcium channel blockers work by inhibiting the slow-channel pathways, or the calcium-dependent channels. As a result, they depress phase 4 depolarization and slow sinoatrial and atrioventricular nodal conduction rates, thus reducing the incidence of paroxysmal supraventricular rhythms (PSVT).
2. Prevention or reduction of supraventricular rhythms
3. Taking phenytoin, an anticonvulsant, along with diltiazem may result in reduced effectiveness of the calcium channel blocker.
4. The physician may prescribe adenosine, which is useful for the treatment of PSVT that has failed to respond to verapamil.

CHAPTER 24
Antianginal Drugs

Chapter Review/Critical Thinking and Application

1. c
2. c
3. a, c, d, e
4. d
5. a
6. b
7. Call 911 and assist the patient until the ambulance arrives. At this time, the nurse does not know the man's condition, and certainly cannot administer someone else's medication to him. Even though isosorbide dinitrate (Novo-Sorbide) is available in a sublingual form, she cannot administer another person's medication, especially to someone with an undetermined condition.
8. Ms. Vickers might be taking a ß-blocker. Fatigue and lethargy are the most common patient complaints with the use of ß-blockers, and mental depression can be exacerbated, particularly in the older adult. Also, one of the central nervous system adverse effects of ß-blockers is the occurrence of unusual dreams.
9. Theresa should always include in her journal a description of the activity she was performing at the time her angina occurred, and the number of tablets she had to take before the pain subsided. Also, she must keep the tablets in an airtight, dark glass bottle away from sunlight, because the active ingredient in nitroglycerin is easily destroyed.

Case Study

1. Chronic stable angina, also known as classic or effort angina, can be triggered by either exertion or stress (cold temperatures or emotions).
2. When experiencing an acute anginal attack, Gideon should take one sublingual tablet as soon as possible after the pain begins, lie down immediately, remain calm, and rest. He can take up to three sublingual tablets every 5 minutes if relief is not experienced after the first tablet.
3. If Gideon experiences no relief after 15 minutes (three sublingual tablets), his handball partner should call 911 and have the emergency response team take him to the hospital. The emergency response team would be better equipped to help him should further complications occur.
4. The ß-blockers are most effective in the treatment of typical exertional angina.

CHAPTER 25
Antihypertensive Drugs

Critical Thinking Crossword

Across
1. Secondary
5. Idiopathic
7. Orthostatic
8. Vasodilators

Down
2. Essential
3. Primary
4. Diuretics
6. ACE

Chapter Review/Critical Thinking and Application

1. c
2. b, d, e
3. c
4. a
5. d

6. Because sodium nitroprusside (Nipride) has a short half-life (10 minutes), the nurses should first discontinue the infusion. Placing Mr. Quester in the Trendelenberg position will also be helpful. Treatment of the hypotension is supportive; pressor drugs can be given to raise the blood pressure quickly if necessary.
7. a. According to the most recent guidelines (see Table 25-1 on p. 464 of the textbook), this patient would be considered prehypertensive.
   b. The patient has "compelling indications," which are conditions that make prehypertension potentially more dangerous for him. To prevent long-term effects, he will be placed on drug therapy for the compelling indications as needed, but will be given no antihypertensive drugs at this time. He will need to be monitored for changes in his blood pressure.
8. a. Captopril (Capoten) is probably best for Irene. In critically ill patients, a drug with a short half-life, such as captopril, is better because if problems arise, they will be short-lived. Also, Irene has liver dysfunction, so captopril has an advantage in that it is not a prodrug. A *prodrug* is inactive in its present form and must be biotransformed in the liver to its active form to be effective.
   b. Because of his history of poor adherence, Kory would benefit from a drug with a long half-life and duration of action, which he would need to take only once a day. Therefore, one of the newer ACE inhibitors, such as benazepril, fosinopril, lisinopril, quinapril, or ramipril, would be best.
9. There is a first-dose effect with prazosin. This means that Mr. Bass will experience a considerable drop in blood pressure after taking the first dose, so he should take it while lying down or before bedtime and arise slowly. This effect decreases with time or with a reduction in the dose as ordered by the physician.
10. a. ß-blockers and ACE inhibitors
    b. Calcium channel blockers and diuretics

Case Study

1. If there are no "compelling indications," initial drug therapy would include thiazide-type diuretics. Other drugs that may also be initiated include ACE inhibitors, angiotensin II receptor blockers, ß-blockers, calcium channel blockers, or a combination. Since John is of African descent, calcium channel blockers would be chosen over ß-blockers and ACE inhibitors.
2. "Compelling indications" are conditions such as heart failure, post–myocardial infarction,

high cardiovascular risk, diabetes mellitus, chronic kidney disease, and recurrent stroke prevention. These conditions, combined with hypertension, may result in eventual organ damage if the hypertension is not controlled. If John has diabetes, then the blood pressure goal would be lower than 130/80 mmHg.
3. He should be taught about the possibility of orthostatic hypotension and taught to change positions slowly, especially after stooping or bending over or when rising from supine or sitting to standing.

CHAPTER 26
Diuretic Drugs

Chapter Review/Critical Thinking and Application

1. c
2. f
3. e
4. i
5. g
6. j
7. h
8. a
9. d
10. b
11. a, c, d, e
12. c
13. a
14. d
15. b
16. a. Ms. Andersen was probably prescribed a carbonic anhydrase inhibitor (CAI).
    b. An undesirable effect of the CAIs is that they elevate the blood glucose level, causing glycosuria in diabetic patients. They may also interact with some oral antihyperglycemic drugs.
17. a. In order for mannitol to be effective in treating acute renal failure, enough kidney blood flow and glomerular filtration must exist to enable the drug to reach the tubules.
    b. Mannitol is always administered intravenously through a filter because it can crystallize when exposed to low temperatures (which is more likely to occur when concentrations exceed 15%).
    c. Arthur's headache and chills are most likely adverse effects of the mannitol therapy. At this time the therapy should be continued, but Arthur should be monitored for the development of more serious adverse effects.
18. a. Mr. Ferrara will be prescribed spironolactone (Aldactone) in high doses; this drug is used often for the treatment of ascites associated with cirrhosis of the liver.

b. His serum potassium level will need to be monitored frequently because he has impaired kidney function.

19. a. Impotence and reduced libido are among the adverse effects of thiazide; Brendan is possibly experiencing these effects.

b. Brendan should stop eating licorice because its consumption can lead to an additive hypokalemia in patients taking thiazide. Brendan's fatigue may be the result of drug toxicity and should be evaluated.

20. It is likely that Mrs. Hill's neighbour was prescribed one of the potassium-sparing diuretics and thus was not instructed to eat additional potassium-rich foods. Mrs. Hill should follow the dietary recommendations provided for her, not for her neighbour.

Case Study

1. These symptoms suggest hypokalemia. Furosemide (Lasix) is a kaliuretic diuretic, which means that potassium is excreted along with sodium and water.

2. Foods high in potassium include bananas, oranges, dates, raisins, plums, fresh vegetables, potatoes (white and sweet), meat, fish, apricots, whole-grain cereals, and legumes.

3. Spironolactone (Aldactone) is a potassium-sparing diuretic. It causes sodium and water to be excreted, but potassium is retained.

4. The combined use of ACE inhibitors or potassium supplements in combination with potassium-sparing diuretics can result in hyperkalemia. When taken together, lithium and potassium-sparing diuretics can result in lithium toxicity. The use of nonsteroidal anti-inflammatory drugs with potassium-sparing diuretics can reduce the effectiveness of the diuretics.

CHAPTER 27
Fluids and Electrolytes

Chapter Review/Critical Thinking and Application

1. a, b, d, e
2. c
3. d
4. c
5. b
6. b
7. **Advantages**: Crystalloids are less expensive than colloids and blood products for replacing fluids and better for emergency short-term plasma volume expansion. They also promote urinary flow. They do not carry the risk of

transmission of viral diseases or anaphylaxis and do not promote bleeding.
Disadvantages: The fluids can leak out of the plasma into the tissues and cells, which results in edema (such as peripheral edema or pulmonary edema). They may dilute plasma proteins, resulting in lower colloid oncotic pressure (COP), and dilute erythrocyte concentration, resulting in decreased oxygen tension. Large volumes are needed to be effective, but prolonged infusions and administration of large volumes may worsen acidosis or alkalosis. Lastly, their effects are relatively short-lived compared with those of colloids.

8. a. Blood products
b. They are the only fluids that contain hemoglobin.
c. They are natural products that require human donors, which means that they can be incompatible with a recipient's immune system; these products can also transmit pathogens from the donor to the recipient.

9. a. Tanya is exhibiting early symptoms of hypokalemia.
b. She should eat foods high in potassium such as bananas, orange juice, and apricots. She may be placed on oral potassium supplements for a short time.

10. a. Hyponatremia
b. Mr. Sanchez can take in sodium by eating foods high in salt such as catsup, mustard, cured meats, and potato chips.
c. Vomiting is a possible adverse effect of oral administration of sodium chloride. If vomiting occurs, Mr. Sanchez needs to be careful about monitoring for further fluid and electrolyte loss.

11. a. Signs of transfusion reaction include apprehension, restlessness, flushed skin, increased pulse and respiration rate, dyspnea, rash, joint or lower back pain, swelling, fever and chills, nausea, weakness, and jaundice.
b. Although it is possible for pathogens such as that causing HIV to be transmitted via blood products, Victor's wife should be reassured that techniques are now used that have drastically reduced the incidence of such problems.
c. Every 15 minutes or more often if needed
d. Victor's restlessness and increased pulse need to be reported to the physician immediately because these are signs of a reaction to the blood product. Have another nurse notify the physician. The nurse should stop the transfusion immediately and change the infusion to normal saline at a

slow rate. Follow the facility's protocol for transfusion reactions.

Case Study

1. The normal total protein level should be 74 g/L. If this level drops below 53 g/L, the colloid oncotic pressure becomes less than the hydrostatic pressure and fluid shifts into the tissues, which results in edema.
2. Colloids increase the colloid oncotic pressure and move fluid from outside the blood vessels to inside the blood vessels, thus reducing the edema.
3. Colloids are the choice for this patient. Crystalloids can leak out of the plasma into the tissues and cells, which results in edema anywhere in the body. Crystalloids also dilute the proteins that are in the plasma, further reducing the colloid oncotic pressure. Finally, crystalloids are more likely to cause edema because of the larger volumes needed to achieve the desired clinical effect. Colloids reduce edema and expand plasma volume by pulling fluid from the extravascular space into the blood vessels.
4. Colloids can alter the coagulation system, which results in impaired coagulation and possible bleeding. They have no oxygen-carrying ability and contain no clotting factors. They may also dilute the plasma protein concentration, which may impair the function of platelets.

CHAPTER 28
Coagulation Modifier Drugs

Chapter Review/Critical Thinking and Application

1. k
2. n
3. j
4. l
5. m
6. b
7. a
8. c
9. i
10. h
11. e
12. g
13. a, c, d
14. b
15. a
16. c
17. b, c, d, e
18. d
19. Yes. The injection site should not be massaged or rubbed before or after the injection because this may cause hematoma formation.

20. a. The anticoagulant effects of heparin can be reversed with protamine sulfate.
    b. In general, 1 mg of protamine can reverse the effects of 100 units of heparin.
    c. The activated partial thromboplastin time is the test most commonly used.
21. If the warfarin (Coumadin) therapy needs to be resumed, resistance is likely to occur because a large dose of vitamin K will maintain its reversal effects for up to 1 week.
22. The physician will probably prescribe one of the antifibrinolytic drugs that are used to stop excessive oozing from surgical sites, such as chest tubes.
23. Desmopressin (DDAVP) is used in patients with type I von Willebrand's disease. It increases the levels of clotting factor VIII.
24. a. No. Alteplase (Activase) is present in the body in a natural state, so it does not induce an antigen–antibody reaction.
    b. Alteplase (Activase) can be readministered because it has a short half-life of 5 minutes. Because of the short half-life, it is given with heparin to prevent reocclusion of the infarcted blood vessel.
25. a. Ursula's symptoms are possible indications of bleeding problems related to the anticoagulation therapy.
    b. Ursula might also be exhibiting a change in pulse rate or rhythm, blood pressure, or level of consciousness.
    c. Notify the physician immediately. Do not administer any other anticoagulants. If Ursula is receiving a continuous infusion, stop the infusion. Prepare to administer the appropriate antidote.

Case Study

1. Use of acetylsalicylic acid (Aspirin) is contraindicated in the presence of peptic ulcer disease. Doug has been started on clopidogrel therapy to reduce the risk of having a stroke.
2. Doug should be taught to watch for signs of abnormal bleeding and should immediately report any of the following signs and symptoms to the health care provider: respiratory difficulty, back pain, skin rash, evidence of gastrointestinal bleeding, any other bleeding abnormality, diarrhea, acute severe headache, and change in vision (blurred vision or loss of vision).
3. Doug needs to take measures to prevent bleeding, such as using a soft toothbrush and an electric razor, and he should take care when trimming his nails, gardening, and participating in rough sports. Doug needs to take precautions

to protect himself from injury and subsequent bleeding or bruising, which can be extremely dangerous while he is taking antiplatelet drugs.

4. Natural health products that contain garlic, ginger, ginseng, and ginkgo should be avoided because they have anticoagulant properties.

CHAPTER 29
Antilipemic Drugs

Chapter Review/Critical Thinking and Application

1. d
2. a, c, d, e
3. a
4. b
5. d
6. c
7. a. Fibric acid derivative; it is believed that these drugs work by activating lipoprotein lipase, an enzyme responsible for the breakdown of cholesterol.
   b. Lipid-lowering drug and vitamin, exact mechanism unknown; beneficial effects are believed to be related to its ability to inhibit lipolysis in adipose tissue, decrease esterification of triglycerides in the liver, and increase the activity of lipase.
   c. HMG-CoA reductase inhibitor; reduces blood cholesterol by decreasing the rate of cholesterol production.
   d. Bile acid sequestrant; binds bile, preventing the resorption of the bile acids from the small intestine. The insoluble bile acid and drug resin complex that is formed is excreted in the feces.
8. Unless Mr. Harris has additional risk factors, his high level of low-density lipoprotein (LDL) cholesterol alone does not warrant drug therapy at this time. All reasonable nonpharmaceutical means of controlling Mr. Harris's LDL level need to be tried and found to fail before he is given drug therapy. Mr. Harris needs to find time in his busy schedule to exercise and eat more wisely.
9. Mr. Jahnke's age and smoking are risk factors, as is the fact that his father died suddenly of heart disease before 55 years of age. Mr. Jahnke's asthma and arthritis are not risk factors, nor is his blood pressure. Mr. Jahnke's high-density lipoprotein (HDL) cholesterol is above 1.6 mmol/L, so it is considered a negative risk factor and can be subtracted from the total number of positive risk factors.
10. Mrs. Kim is experiencing constipation and belching associated with cholestyramine (Novo-Cholamine) use (she may also be experiencing

heartburn, nausea, and bloating). Mrs. Kim requires extra patient teaching and support to help her maintain adherence to the drug therapy. She should be assured that these adverse effects will probably diminish over time.

11. No. Justus is not a candidate for niacin therapy for two reasons: (1) niacin is not recommended with lovastatin because it can lead to the development of rhabdomyolysis, and (2) niacin use is contraindicated in patients with peptic ulcer.
12. Mrs. Nguyen must take her antihypertensive and cholestyramine (Novo-Cholamine) at different times of the day because the bile acid sequestrant may interfere significantly with the absorption of other drugs taken at the same time. All other drugs should be taken at least 1 hour before or 4 to 6 hours after the administration of antilipemics. Cholestyramine should be taken just before or with meals. Also, the powder form of cholestyramine should be allowed to dissolve slowly in at least 60 mL of fluid, without stirring, for at least 1 minute. Stirring causes the powder to clump. The powder may not mix totally in the glass and more fluid may need to be added to the glass. The powder may also be mixed thoroughly with food, such as crushed pineapple.

Case Study

1. No, Mr. Miller is not right. Dietary measures are a part of antilipemic therapy. Nonpharmacological measures include consumption of a low-fat low-cholesterol diet; supervised, moderate exercise; weight loss; cessation of smoking or drinking; and relaxation therapy.
2. Atorvastatin (Lipitor) is used primarily to lower total and LDL cholesterol as well as triglyceride levels. It has been shown to raise the HDL level as well.
3. Elevations in liver enzyme levels may also occur and the patient should be monitored for excessive elevations, which may indicate the need for alternative drug therapy. In addition, total cholesterol level, LDL/HDL cholesterol levels, and triglyceride levels need to be monitored to evaluate therapeutic effect.
4. Myopathy (muscle pain) is an uncommon but clinically important adverse effect that may occur in some patients taking statins. It may progress to a serious condition known as *rhabdomyolysis* in which the breakdown of muscle protein occurs, leading to myoglobinuria and possible kidney damage. Patients receiving statin therapy should be taught to report unexplained muscle pain to their health care provider immediately.

CHAPTER 30
Pituitary Drugs

Chapter Review/Critical Thinking and Application

1. a. Glucocorticoids, mineralocorticoids, androgens
   b. cosyntropin
   c. Regulates anabolic processes related to growth and adaptation to stressors; promotes skeletal and muscle growth; increases protein synthesis; increases liver glycogenolysis; increases fat mobilization
   d. somatropin (Humatrope) and octreotide (Sandostatin)
   e. Antidiuretic hormone
   f. vasopressin and desmopressin
   g. Promotes uterine contractions
   h. oxytocin
2. b, e, f
3. d
4. b
5. d
6. c
7. a. Alexis might well benefit from administration of cosyntropin not only to treat the pain associated with inflammation but also to produce increased comfort and muscle strength.
   b. Cautions include checking to see whether Alexis may be pregnant or nursing. Contraindications to cosyntropin use include osteoporosis, heart failure, peptic ulcer disease, hypertension, recent surgery, and dysfunction of the adrenocortex. Drug interactions of which the nurse should be mindful are interactions with amphotericin B (Amphotec) and drugs that lower potassium level, such as some diuretics.
   c. Other parameters to assess include baseline levels of vital signs, electrolyte values, blood glucose levels, chest radiographic findings, complete blood count results, intake and output, daily weight, and cortisol levels.
   d. Patient teaching plans should include issues listed at length in the Patient Education box in this chapter.
8. In addition to information about proper subcutaneous injection techniques, the teaching plan should include a reminder of the dosage form and amount and the importance of adherence to therapy. The parents should be shown how to keep a journal of Patricia's growth measurements.
9. Contraindications to the use of growth hormone somatropin include closed epiphyseal plates of the

long bones. Jack should not receive the medication simply to get taller but only when diagnosed with an appropriate medical condition and then only if he has not stopped growing. Chances are that at age 25 he has stopped growing.

Case Study

1. Mr. Collins will probably be found to have diabetes insipidus; if so, he will benefit from treatment with vasopressin or desmopressin.
2. Assessment strategies should include evaluating pulse, vital signs, intake and output, daily weight, and edema. Desmopressin should be given cautiously in patients with chronic migraines, seizures, and asthma.
3. Treatment will be via nasal spray, 1 to 2 sprays administered into each nostril twice daily. This should increase water resorption in the distal tubules and collecting ducts of the nephron, performing all the physiological functions of antidiuretic hormone.
4. It should eliminate Mr. Collins's severe thirst and decrease his urinary output.

CHAPTER 31
Thyroid and Antithyroid Drugs

Critical Thinking Crossword

Across
3. Secondary
6. Thyroxine
7. Primary

Down
1. Levothyroxine
2. Hyperthyroidism
4. Propylthiouracil
5. Tertiary
6. Thyrotropin

Chapter Review/Critical Thinking and Application

1. c
2. d
3. a
4. a, c, d
5. c
6. Mrs. de Andrade probably has hypothyroidism, which may result in the formation of a goitre, an enlargement of the thyroid gland resulting from its overstimulation by elevated levels of thyroid-stimulating hormone. She may benefit from one of the thyroid agents, including thyroid, thyroglobulin, levothyroxine (Eltroxin), or liothyronine. Levothyroxine is

generally preferred because as a chemically pure formulation of 100% thryroxine, its hormonal content is standardized; therefore, its effect is predictable.

7. Even if it can be determined that the last several symptoms are due to menopause, the combination of the rest of the symptoms, plus Ms. Hilton's history, indicate the strong possibility that she has hyperthyroidism. This is especially worth investigating since it is often caused by Graves' disease.

8. Surgery to remove all or part of the thyroid gland is an effective way to treat hyperthyroidism, but as a result, lifelong hormone replacement is normally required.

Case Study

1. Goldie's symptoms suggest hypothyroidism. A thyroid replacement hormone, such as levothyroxine, would be indicated for this condition.

2. The thyroid preparations are given to replace what the thyroid gland cannot itself produce in order to achieve normal thyroid levels, known as *euthyroid* condition.

3. Thyroid preparations should be taken at the same time every day to maintain constant blood levels. Taking the medication in the morning will help reduce problems with insomnia, which may result when the medication is taken later in the day or in the evening.

CHAPTER 32
Antidiabetic Drugs

Chapter Review/Critical Thinking and Application

1. b
2. d
3. a
4. c
5. c
6. b
7. 4.9 units of insulin (13.2 mmol – 8.3 mmol = 4.9)
8. Sitagliptin (Januvia) is indicated in combination with metformin in adult patients with type 2 diabetes mellitus to improve glycemic control when diet and exercise and use of metformin do not provide adequate control. Sitagliptin is a highly selective inhibitor of the dipeptidyl peptidase 4 (DPP-4) enzyme that enhances incretin hormones. The incretin hormones are released by the intestine throughout the day, and levels increased in response to a meal are part of an endogenous system involved in the physiological regulation

of glucose homeostasis. Consequently, treatment with sitagliptin improves β-cell responsiveness to glucose and stimulates insulin release.

9. a. Alice's diet should include a high intake of protein and a low intake of carbohydrates.
   b. The brain requires a constant supply of glucose to function. Thus, the central nervous system manifestations of hypoglycemia (such as irritability) are often the first to appear.
   c. In the conscious person, oral forms of glucose are used, such as rapidly dissolving buccal tablets or semisolid gel forms designed for rapid mucosal absorption. She could also try corn syrup, honey, fruit juice, a nondiet soft drink, or a small snack such as crackers or half a sandwich.

10. a. Bill should check the order at least three times and have another registered nurse check the prepared injection to be sure it is in accordance with the physician's order.
    b. The nurse, of course. Humulin-R is regular insulin and regular insulin is clear in appearance.
    c. If left at room temperature, the insulin should have been used within 1 month; otherwise, it should have been refrigerated.

11. a. Alec requires an intermediate-acting insulin.
    b. Alec's religious beliefs might prohibit him from using insulin made from pork. Because of the availability of human biosynthetic and analogue insulins, Alec should not need to use any insulins containing pork.

12. a. Mrs. Franklin needs to make some significant lifestyle changes. She must stop smoking, lose weight, and exercise regularly, which will help with both the high blood glucose level and the hypertension.
    b. Mrs. Franklin should continue with her exercise and weight loss program; however, because her blood glucose level is still elevated, she also requires an oral antidiabetic drug.

13. a. Hypoglycemia
    b. Dennis may have been drinking alcohol. Sulfonylureas may interact with alcohol in a way that is similar to the interaction with disulfiram, which is used to deter alcohol ingestion in persons with chronic alcoholism. This *disulfiram-type* reaction includes vomiting and hypertension.

14. a. 20 units of NPH (Novolin ge NPH) insulin plus 4 units regular insulin
    b. No coverage
    c. 6 units of regular insulin

Case Study

1. The second-generation sulfonylureas have many advantages over the older agents, including much greater potency. Also, chlorpropamide (Novo-Propamide) is dependent on the kidneys for elimination and can cause toxicity in patients with decreased renal function. Gliclazide (Diamicron) use is not contraindicated in patients with severe kidney failure.
2. Gliclazide has a rapid onset of action; its effect is thus much like the body's normal response to meals when greater levels of insulin are rapidly required to deal with the increased glucose in the blood.
3. Gliclazide works best if given 30 minutes before meals.
4. Mr. Dressel should contact his physician immediately. He may require a change in his diabetic treatment while he is sick because vomiting and inability to eat can cause a change in his blood glucose levels.

CHAPTER 33
Adrenal Drugs

Chapter Review/Critical Thinking and Application

1. a
2. c
3. a, b, c
4. b
5. d
6. c
7. Ms. Rivera's glucocorticoid can interact with acetylsalicytic acid (Aspirin) and other nonsteroidal anti-inflammatory drugs (NSAIDs), producing additive effects. Also, she should avoid persons with infections because her own immune system is suppressed. The children in the hospital may have infections. In addition, she should report any fever, increased weakness and lethargy, or sore throat.
8. a. The use of systemic glucocorticoids with antidiabetic agents may reduce the hypoglycemic effect of those drugs. A baseline blood glucose level should be determined and Peter should be monitored for any problems.
   b. Oral systemic adrenal agents should be taken with milk, food, or nonsystemic antacids (such as aluminum-, calcium-, or magnesium-containing antacids), unless contraindicated, to minimize gastrointestinal upset. Another option is for the physician to order a histamine-2 receptor antagonist

or proton pump inhibitors to prevent ulcer formation (glucocorticoids may cause gastric ulcers). Patients should be encouraged *not* to take the drug with alcohol, acetylsalicytic acid (Aspirin), or other NSAIDs to minimize gastric irritation and gastric bleeding.
9. Intervene. The student nurse should, while wearing gloves, apply the medication with a sterile tongue depressor or cotton-tipped applicator if the skin is intact. If the skin is not intact, a sterile technique should be used.
10. In addition to routine teaching about inhaler administration technique, Nina should be instructed to rinse with lukewarm water after using the inhaler, to prevent the development of an oral fungal infection.

Case Study

1. Administration of prednisone causes the body to stop producing hormones; tapering the dose allows the body time to start making it again. Sudden discontinuation of these drugs can precipitate an adrenal crisis caused by a sudden drop in the serum levels of cortisone. Also, a short term of therapy will reduce the effects that often occur with long-term therapy.
2. Short- or long-term therapy may cause steroid psychosis. In addition, long-term effects cause cushingoid symptoms, including moon face, weight gain, muscle wasting, and increased deposition of fat in the trunk area, leading to truncal obesity.
3. Glucocorticoid. Biological functions of glucocorticoids include anti-inflammatory actions, maintenance of normal blood pressure, carbohydrate and protein metabolism, fat metabolism, and stress effects. Biological functions of mineralocorticoids include sodium and water resorption, blood pressure control, and potassium levels and pH of blood.
4. The best time for Cheri to take this drug is early in the morning (0600 to 0900) because this results in the least amount of adrenal suppression.

CHAPTER 34
Women's Health Drugs

Chapter Review/Critical Thinking and Application

1. b, c, d, e
2. a
3. a
4. b

5. b
6. c, e, f
7. a. Ask Isabelle if she is taking medication for depression. Estrogen therapy is indicated for the symptoms of menopause, but the use of estrogen with a tricyclic antidepressant may result in toxicity of the latter drug.
    b. The smallest dose of estrogen that alleviates the symptoms is used for the shortest possible time.
8. a. The physician will probably prescribe medroxyprogesterone, which is indicated for treatment of secondary amenorrhea.
    b. Ms. Boutrimas's dose of antidiabetic drug may need to be adjusted because of a possible decrease in glucose tolerance when progestins and antidiabetic drugs are taken together.
9. a. Perhaps Jacklyn's prescription could be switched to a 28-day form of norethindrone/ethinyl estradiol, which is taken for all 28 days of the menstrual cycle rather than for 3 weeks with 1 week off.
    b. One of the benefits of oral contraceptive use is decreased blood loss during menstruation.
10. a. Choriogonadotropin-alfa is often given in a carefully timed fashion after follicle-stimulating hormone–active therapy with a drug such as mentropin or clomiphene, when patient monitoring indicates insufficient maturation of ovarian follicles. Once the ovaries have been sufficiently stimulated (with 9 to 12 days of therapy), then a single large dose of choriogonadotropin-alfa is given the next day.
    b. This course of drugs may be repeated a second and third time if needed.
11. Mrs. Ingalls needs to know that smoking can diminish the therapeutic effects of the estrogen she is taking and can add to the risk of thrombosis. Also, she should be cautioned to wear sunscreen while in Aruba because estrogen makes the skin more susceptible to sunburn.
12. a. Mrs. Vu is assuming that the medication is estrogen therapy. Alendronate (Fosamax) is indicated to prevent osteoporosis in postmenopausal women. The nurse will need to explain to her that it is the first nonestrogen, nonhormonal medication used for prevention of bone loss in the early postmenopausal period; for women who experience early menopause, the dose of 5 mg daily is recommended.
    b. Mrs. Vu experienced early menopause; other risk factors associated with the development

of postmenopausal osteoporosis include thin body build, Caucasian or Asian race, family history of osteoporosis, and moderately low bone mass. She would need to be assessed for these other risk factors.

Case Study

1. The nonpharmacological treatment of premature labour includes bed rest, sedation, and hydration. Ms. O'Hara should be placed in the left lateral recumbent position to minimize hypotension and increase blood flow to the kidneys and blood flow to the fetus.
2. In theory, tocolytic drugs are used to delay premature labour for up to 48 hours in order to gain time to allow steroids to hasten fetal lung development. One example of a tocolytic drug is ritodrine, a β_2-adrenergic agonist, which relaxes the uterus by stimulating the β_2-adrenergic receptors of the uterine muscle, resulting in a decrease in the intensity and frequency of uterine contractions. Ritodine was removed from the Canadian market because of adverse effects of maternal pulmonary edema. Magnesium sulfate acts as competitive antagonist to calcium entry into the myocyte, resulting in decreased myometrial contractility. However, the use of tocolytics has not reduced the risk of preterm or low birth weight births or improved neonatal outcomes. In addition, tocolytics are associated with maternal adverse effects. Health Canada has not approved any drug for use as a tocolytic.

CHAPTER 35
Men's Health Drugs

Chapter Review/Critical Thinking and Application

1. b
2. b, d, f
3. a
4. d
5. c
6. a
7. a. Testosterone's poor performance in the oral dose form is due to the fact that most of a dose is metabolized and destroyed by the liver before it can reach the circulation, known as the *first-pass effect*. Unlike other oral testosterone preparations, testosterone undecanoate (Andriol) is able to bypass the liver via the lymphatic system and is therefore orally bioavailable. Therapy with testosterone undecanoate increases plasma levels of testosterone and its active

metabolites, leading to a regular therapeutic effect.

b. Contraindications that could apply to Mr. Michaels include significant heart, liver, or kidney dysfunction; breast carcinoma; or known or suspected prostate cancer.

8. a. With actuated metered-dose pumps, each forced depression (actuation) of the pump will expel a specific (metered) dose of drug through a mouthpiece (the actuator). The label "60 actuation metered-dose" means the pump can be depressed 60 times, delivering 1.25 g of gel per actuation, for a total of 75 g of gel (the product usually has 88 g to take into account priming; see *b*, below). Mr. Koo should therefore be careful to note how many times he is pumping the canister in order to get the right dosage of testosterone, which would usually be 5 g of gel (equivalent to 50 mg of testosterone) per day.

b. The metered-dose AndroGel pump has to be primed prior to use; this usually takes about five depressions to remove the air, followed by gel discharge. The initial two gel discharges should be discarded so that an accurate gel dose is delivered. Mr. Koo should be especially careful when discarding the waste gel, to make sure other household members do not accidentally eat or touch it, especially since he is living with two small children.

9. a. Finasteride (Proscar) works by inhibiting the enzymatic process responsible for converting testosterone to 5α-dihydrotestosterone (DHT), which is the principal androgen responsible for stimulating prostatic growth. It can dramatically lower the prostatic DHT concentrations, thereby reducing testosterone concentrations and causing the hypertrophied prostate to decrease in size.

b. Mr. Olafson's teaching plan should include the rationale for therapy and a full disclosure of adverse effects.

10. The patch is contained in a pouch that should be applied immediately after opening the pouch and removing the protective release liner. The patch should be pressed firmly in place, making sure there is good contact with the skin, especially around the edges. The adhesive side of the Androderm patch should be applied to a clean, dry area of the skin on the back, abdomen, upper arms, or thighs. Bony prominences, such as the shoulder and hip areas, should be avoided. It should not be applied to the scrotum. The sites of application should be rotated, with an interval of 7 days between applications to the same site. The area selected should not be oily, damaged, or irritated.

Case Study

1. Sildenafil (Viagra) should be used cautiously in patients with renal disorders, hypertension, diabetes, and cardiovascular disease, and it is contraindicated if Mr. Ang is taking nitrates because of the danger for severe hypotensive effects.

2. Headache, dizziness, flushing, and dyspepsia are the most common adverse effects reported. In addition, sildenafil is highly protein bound and may interact with many drugs. Mr. Ang should check with the doctor before taking any other medication.

3. Older individuals experience declining liver function, so drugs may not be metabolized as effectively as when they were younger. In addition, there have been reports of vision loss in men who have been taking this class of drug.

4. Sildenafil should be taken 1 hour before intercourse.

CHAPTER 36
Antihistamines, Decongestants, Antitussives, and Expectorants

Chapter Review/Critical Thinking and Application

1. a, b, c
2. a
3. b
4. c
5. b
6. d
7. The histamine-1 (H_1) blockers cannot push off histamine that is already bound to its receptor. Because they compete with histamine for unoccupied receptors, they work best when given early in a reaction, before all of the histamine can bind to receptors.
8. Yes. The traditional antihistamines have anticholinergic effects, which may make them more effective in some cases. Patients respond to and tolerate these agents quite well. Also, because many traditional antihistamines are generically available, they are often much less expensive.
9. No. Mrs. Ling is likely experiencing rebound congestion caused by sustained use of the oxymetazoline HCl (Afrin Sinus and Allergy) for several days.
10. Keith is exhibiting symptoms of the cardiovascular effects that can occur when a

topically applied adrenergic nasal decongestant is somewhat absorbed into the bloodstream.

11. Dextromethorphan (Benylin)'s mechanism of action is the same as that of the other drugs. It suppresses the cough reflex through direct action on the cough centre in the central nervous system (medulla). It also provides analgesia and has a drying effect on the mucosa of the respiratory tract, which also increases the viscosity of respiratory secretions. This helps to reduce such symptoms as runny nose and postnasal drip. However, because it is not an opioid, it does not have analgesic properties, nor does it cause addiction or central nervous system depression. Dextromethorphan may potentiate the serotonergic effects of MAOIs, and thus concurrent administration is contraindicated.

12. He should ask Irene whether she is taking any thyroid medication. A drug interaction (an additive hypothyroid effect) can occur if she takes an expectorant with an antithyroid drug. Irene should call her health care provider before she goes to the drugstore.

13. First, Lisa's brother received Robitussin A-C, a narcotic antitussive containing codeine, for his cough. Lisa has been prescribed Robitussin, an expectorant, for her nonproductive cough associated with acute bronchitis. Second, even if the two children were prescribed the same drug, Lisa is only 5 years old and requires a smaller dosage than her brother.

14. Some decongestants have stimulating effects on the cardiac and central nervous system that may result in palpitations, insomnia, restlessness, and nervousness. Justin should avoid caffeine and caffeine-containing products to avoid further excessive central nervous system stimulation.

Case Study

1. James's diabetes should not affect his treatment.
2. The topical diphenhydramine (Anti-Itch Cream) might come in combination with a drug such as calamine, camphor, or zinc oxide.
3. James should be informed that taking any of the sedating antihistamines may precipitate drowsiness and thus he should should be told to avoid driving or operating heavy machinery should these adverse effects occur or until he knows how he will respond to the medication.
4. James should also be informed not to consume alcohol or take other central nervous system depressants because they may interact with the diphenhydramine to exacerbate drowsiness and sedation.

CHAPTER 37
Bronchodilators and Other Respiratory Drugs

Chapter Review/Critical Thinking and Application

1. b, d, e, f
2. d
3. d
4. b
5. c
6. a
7. The three main etiological factors of asthma are predisposing, causal, and contributing.
8. Tom is exhibiting some adverse effects of theophylline therapy and the level in his blood is probably too high (the common therapeutic range for theophylline in the blood is 55 to 110 micromoles/L). Tom may require a reduction in dosage.
9. The nurse needs to know how much Willie weighs. The dosage of subcutaneous epinephrine is 0.01 to 0.03 mg/kg q5 min prn.
10. Sylvia is exhibiting dose-related adverse effects of the salbutamol (Ventolin), possibly because she used it too frequently. Sylvia needs to be reminded to use her medication exactly as prescribed.
11. a. Anticholinergics, corticosteroids, and ß-agonists
    b. Of concern is Mrs. Di Risio's glaucoma. Use of ipratropium bromide (an anticholinergic) is contraindicated in patients with glaucoma, and corticosteroids should be used with caution in patients with glaucoma.
12. a. The disadvantage to administering the corticosteroids orally is that they can then have systemic effects, such as adrenocortical insufficiency, increased susceptibility to infection, fluid and electrolyte disturbances, endocrine effects, dermatological effects, and nervous system effects. They can also interact with other systemically administered drugs. (The advantage to administering corticosteroids by inhalation is that their action is limited to the topical site of action—the lungs. In that way, they have no systemic effects and cannot interact with other systemically administered drugs.)
    b. Yes. The use of an inhaled corticosteroid frequently allows a reduction in the daily dose of the systemic corticosteroid. This reduction should be gradual.
13. a. Advair contains fluticasone propionate, a corticosteroid, and salmeterol xinaforte, a long-acting bronchodilator. Advair is used for the maintenance treatment of asthma.

b. To relieve acute asthmatic symptoms, Sam should use a rapid-onset, short-duration inhaled bronchodilator (e.g., salbutamol).

Case Study

1. These drugs are not direct bronchodilators; they work to reduce the inflammatory response in the lungs.
2. They are primarily used for oral prophylaxis and chronic treatment of asthma and are not recommended for treatment of acute asthma attacks.
3. There are no interactions between ibuprofen and montelukast; however, Jennie should continue to check with her physician before taking other over-the-counter medications.
4. These agents should be taken every night on a continuous schedule, even if symptoms improve.

CHAPTER 38
Antibiotics Part 1: Sulfonamides, Penicillins, Cephalosporins, Macrolides, and Tetracyclines

Critical Thinking Crossword

Across
3. Prophylactic
6. tetracycline
7. Penicillin
8. Bactericidal
9. cephalosporin

Down
1. Macrolide
2. Sulfonamide
4. Bacteriostatic
5. Superinfection

Chapter Review/Critical Thinking and Application

1. b, d, e
2. a
3. b
4. c
5. d
6. c
7. Cefoxitin is frequently used in patients undergoing abdominal or colorectal surgeries because it can kill intestinal bacteria such as gram-positive, gram-negative, and anaerobic bacteria.
8. a. Sean should not take the doxycycline (Doxycin) with milk because that can result in a significant reduction in the oral absorption of the drug. Sean should

also be aware that tetracyclines can cause photosensitivity. He should stay out of the sun.
   b. The diarrhea is probably the result of alteration of the intestinal flora caused by the drug therapy.
9. Sandra is experiencing a superinfection because the antibiotics that she has been taking for the bronchitis have reduced the normal vaginal bacterial flora, and the yeast that is usually kept in balance by this normal flora has an opportunity to grow and cause an infection.

Case Study

1. This patient should be assessed for severe hepatitis, glomerular nephritis, and uremia. Also, the use of sulfamethoxazole trimethoprim (Protrin) is contraindicated in cases of known drug allergy to sulfonamides or chemically related drugs such as sulfonylureas (used for diabetes), thiazide and loop diuretics, and carbonic anhydrase inhibitors.
2. If he is taking a sulfonylurea for the type 2 diabetes, close monitoring is needed because sulfonamides can potentiate the hypoglycemic effects of sulfonylureas in diabetes. In addition, even though he is currently receiving intravenous heparin and not warfarin, he may be placed on oral anticoagulants soon, so the nurse should should keep in mind that sulfonamides can potentiate the anticoagulant effects of warfarin and lead to hemorrhage.
3. These antibiotics achieve high concentrations in the kidneys, through which they are eliminated. Therefore, they are primarily used in the treatment of urinary tract infections.
4. Sulfonamides do not actually destroy bacteria but inhibit their growth. For this reason, they are considered bacteriostatic antibiotics. Bactericidal antibiotics kill bacteria.

CHAPTER 39
Antibiotics Part 2: Aminoglycosides, Fluoroquinolones, and Other Drugs

Chapter Review/Critical Thinking and Application

1. c
2. b
3. a, b, c, d
4. a
5. The current practice is once-a-day aminoglycoside dosing. The nurses can explain to Angie that studies have shown that once-daily dosing provides a sufficient plasma drug

concentartion to kill bacteria and also has equal or lower risk of toxicity compared with multiple-daily dosing. Hopefully, this type of dosing will be safer and more effective for Angie.

6. A blood sample for measurement of "trough" level is drawn at least 18 hours after a dose is administered (24 hours if the patient has kidney impairment). The therapeutic goal is a trough level of at or below 1 mcg/mL. If the trough level is above 2 mcg/mL, then the patient is at greater risk for ototoxicity and nephrotoxicity. Trough levels should be monitored once every 3 days until the drug is stopped. In addition, kidney function is monitored by measuring serum creatinine levels. A rising serum creatinine suggests reduced creatinine clearance by the kidneys. Serum creatinine level should be measured at least twice weekly.

7. Yes. In patients who receive amiodarone therapy, dangerous cardiac dysrhythmias are more likely to occur when quinolones are taken. Another drug besides levofloxacin may show effectiveness against the bacteria that is causing the infection.

8. Nitrofurantoin (Macrodantin) is used primarily to treat urinary tract infections because it is excreted via the kidneys and concentrates in the urine. It can cause significant kidney impairment but is usually well tolerated if the patient is kept well hydrated. The rationale behind forcing fluids is to facilitate the elimination of the drug. Consequently, the drug will exert its desired effect and the patient will not be at risk for kidney damage.

Case Study

1. Ototoxicity and nephrotoxicity. Symptoms of ototoxicity include dizziness, tinnitus, and hearing loss. Symptoms of nephrotoxicity include urinary casts, proteinuria, and increased blood urea nitrogen and serum creatinine levels. Keeping the drug blood levels (peak and trough) within a specific therapeutic range can help prevent those toxicities.

2. The aminoglycosides and penicillins are often used together because they have a synergistic effect; that is, the combined effect of the two drugs is greater than that of either drug alone.

3. There is certainly a concern. The desired trough level is 1 mcg/mL, so a level of 3 mcg/mL could mean that Virgil is receiving a dose that is too high. The increased serum creatinine level is also a concern because it could be an

indication of impaired kidney function. The physician should be notified immediately and doses of the aminoglycoside withheld until the physician responds.

CHAPTER 40
Antiviral Drugs

Chapter Review/Critical Thinking and Application

1. d
2. d
3. a
4. c
5. a, b
6. Any drug that kills a virus can also kill healthy cells. Viruses must enter cells to replicate. Therefore, antiviral drugs must also enter the host cells. Few drugs can kill only the virus and leave the body's cells unharmed. Viruses are also difficult to kill because often by the time they are discovered, they have finished replicating. At that point, it is too late for antiviral agents, which interfere with viral replication, to work.
7. Yes. Zidovudine (Retrovir [AZT]), one of the few anti-HIV drugs known to prolong patient survival, can be used for maternal and fetal treatment. Between 14 and 34 weeks of pregnancy, Amy can receive oral zidovudine capsules. During labour she can receive zidovudine intravenously. Oral drug therapy (syrup) for the infant can begin within 12 hours of delivery and continue for 6 weeks. However, transmission to infants may still occur in some cases despite the use of this regimen.
8. a. Acyclovir (Zovirax) is indicated for the varicella-zoster virus (shingles). The greatest benefit occurs when treatment is initiated within 48 hours of the onset of lesions.
   b. Bailey's daily fluid intake should be at least 2400 mL while she is taking acyclovir. Also, acyclovir capsules may be taken with food.
   c. Bailey can be treated with acyclovir again; it is the drug of choice for treatment of both initial and recurrent episodes of shingles.
9. a. Ribavirin (Virazole) is used to treat infections caused by respiratory syncytial virus.
   b. Yes. Brenda's treatment will last at least 3 days but not more than 7 days. Treatment with ribavirin should be started as soon as possible within the first 3 days of an infection with respiratory syncytial virus.
10. a. The patient may be experiencing zidovudine's major dose-limiting adverse effect, which is bone marrow suppression.

b. Eduardo should mix the powder solution in at least 115 mL of water, not fruit juice or juice containing acid, and drink it immediately. The drug should be taken on an empty stomach 1 hour before meals or 2 hours after meals.

c. No. Antacids taken concurrently with didanosine can cause increased absorption of the didanosine, which is a positive effect.

11. No. The nurse's co-worker is doing fine. Acyclovir administered by intravenous infusion is first diluted in sterile water or in a solution recommended by the manufacturer and is administered slowly over at least 1 hour.

12. No. Therapy with oseltamivir (Tamiflu) should begin within 2 days of the onset of influenza. It is probably too late for this drug to be effective for Stacey.

Case Study

1. Mr. Cuomo should wear a glove or finger cot when applying topical acyclovir (Zovirax) to the affected area, which should be kept clean and dry. Also, he should not use any other creams or ointments on the area.

2. Mr. Cuomo's herpes cannot be "cured," although the acyclovir will help manage the symptoms.

3. Stress the importance of treatment for Mr. Cuomo and his sexual partner, and discuss with him how to prevent transmission of the virus.

4. There are several viruses in the *Herpesviridae* family, including herpes simplex type 1 (HSV-1), which causes mucocutaneous herpes, usually blisters around the mouth; varicella-zoster virus (herpes simplex type 3, or HSV-3), which causes both chickenpox and shingles; herpesvirus type 4 (also called Epstein-Barr virus or EBV); and herpesvirus type 8, which is believed by some to cause Kaposi's sarcoma, a cancer associated with AIDS.

CHAPTER 41
Antituberculosis Drugs

Chapter Review/Critical Thinking and Application

1. a
2. b
3. a, b, c
4. c
5. a
6. a. Liver function studies should be performed because isoniazid can cause liver impairment. A complete blood count, including hemoglobulin and hematocrit value, should be checked because of the hematological disorders isoniazid can cause.

b. Diane may be a slow acetylator. Acetylation, the process by which isoniazid is metabolized in the liver, requires certain enzymes to break down the isoniazid. In slow acetylators, who have a genetic deficiency of the enzymes, the isoniazid accumulates. The dosage of isoniazid may need to be adjusted downward in these patients.

7. a. Streptomycin is administered intramuscularly, deep in a large muscle mass, and the sites are rotated.

b. The adverse effects of streptomycin are ototoxicity and nephrotoxicity.

c. Although it may not be a concern in terms of Ms. Innes's streptomycin therapy, oral contraceptives become ineffective when given with rifampin. If rifampin is part of her therapy, Ms. Innes should switch to another form of birth control.

8. A thorough eye examination may be called for before the institution of therapy because ethambutol can cause a decrease in visual acuity resulting from optic neuritis, which is also a contraindication to the use of ethambutol.

9. a. Mr. Fiore needs to know that his adherence to therapy is essential for achieving a cure. Although he is keeping his follow-up appointments, Mr. Fiore also needs to take his medication as ordered. He should be warned to not consume alcohol, and he should be encouraged to take care of himself with adequate nutrition, rest, and relaxation.

b. The therapeutic response can be confirmed by results of laboratory studies (sputum culture and sensitivity tests) and chest radiographic findings.

10. a. Frannie, as with all patients taking antituberculosis drugs, needs to be adherent to the therapy and keep her follow-up appointments. She should be reminded that she can spread the disease (during the initial period of the illness); she should wash her hands frequently and cover her mouth when coughing or sneezing. Frannie also needs adequate nutrition and rest.

b. It is likely that Frannie is on rifampin therapy. She should be told that her urine, stool, saliva, sputum, sweat, or tears may become red-orange-brown and that this is an effect of rifampin therapy.

Case Study

1. George's gout is a consideration; pyrazinamide (Tebrazid) can cause hyperuricemia, so gout or flare-ups of gout can occur in susceptible patients. His diabetes is a concern as well; ethambutol (Etibi) should be used cautiously in patients with diabetes. A baseline hearing test should be performed if streptomycin is considered because this drug may cause ototoxicity.

2. An individual with a genetic deficiency of the liver enzymes that metabolize drugs can be classified as a "slow acetylator." When isoniazid is taken by slow acetylators, the drug accumulates because there is not enough of the enzymes to break down the isoniazid. As a result, the dosage of isoniazid may need to be reduced.

3. Results of liver function tests should be assessed carefully before therapy is initiated, because some drugs (isoniazid [Dom Isoniazid], pyrazinamide) are heptatotoxic. Liver function test results should be monitored closely during therapy as well.

4. Patients should take pyridoxine (vitamin B$_6$) as prescribed by the physician to prevent some of the neurological adverse effects of isoniazid, such as peripheral neuritis.

CHAPTER 42
Antifungal Drugs

Chapter Review/Critical Thinking and Application

1. j
2. e
3. f
4. g
5. a
6. c
7. h
8. i
9. d
10. b
11. c
12. b, c, e
13. d
14. b
15. a
16. Mycotic infections are difficult to treat and research into new drugs has occurred at a slow pace, in part because the necessary chemical concentrations of the experimental agents cannot be tolerated by humans.

17. a. Fluconazole (Diflucan), unlike itraconazole (Sporanox), can pass into the cerebrospinal fluid, making it effective in the treatment of cryptococcal meningitis. It is considered to be the most effective of the imidazoles for treating several infections.
    b. Unfortunately, Mr. Kim will need to remain on a reduced dosage of the medication for 10 to 12 weeks after the negative results of the cerebrospinal fluid culture.

18. a. The amphotericin B (Fungizone) should be diluted according to the manufacturer's guidelines. Sterile water without a bacteriostatic agent (such as benzyl alcohol, which may cause precipitation of the antibiotic) is recommended for its reconstitution, and 5% dextrose in water may be used for infusion. Amphotericin B is administered by *slow* intravenous infusion over 2 to 6 hours.
    b. Fever, chills, hypotension, tachycardia, malaise, muscle and joint pain, anorexia, nausea and vomiting, and headache are possible adverse effects.
    c. No. Almost all patients experience these effects. To decrease their severity, James may be pretreated with an antipyretic (e.g., acetaminophen), an antihistamine, and an antiemetic.

19. Lewis should be aware that he will be taking the medication for 2 to 6 weeks, until the infection clears. During that time, he should avoid alcohol because of the increased risk for hepatoxicity and he should take the medication with food to avoid gastrointestinal upset. Ketoconazole (Nu-Ketocon) also causes photophobia, so Lewis should avoid the sun or use sunscreen and sunglasses with ultraviolet protection.

Case Study

1. Voriconazole (Vfend) is used for major fungal infections in patients who do not tolerate or respond to other antifungal agents.

2. The use of voriconazole is contraindicated in patients taking other drugs that are metabolized by the cytochrome P-450 enzyme 3A4 (e.g., quinidine), because of the risk of inducing serious cardiac dysrhythmias.

3. Careful cardiac monitoring should be done if Sally is taking quinidine while taking voriconazole.

CHAPTER 43
Antimalarial, Antiprotozoal, and Anthelmintic Drugs

Chapter Review/Critical Thinking and Application

1. a
2. b
3. c
4. b, e
5. d
6. c
7. Malaria is caused by *Plasmodium* organisms. During the asexual stage of the *Plasmodium* life cycle, which occurs in the human host, the parasite resides for a short time outside the erythrocyte. This is called the *exoerythrocytic phase*. The most effective agent for eradicating the parasite during this phase is primaquine.
8. Before primaquine is administered, Professor Henson should be given a pregnancy test. This is a pregnancy category C agent, so the nurse will need to know if certain precautions are needed in Professor Henson's case. She should also be assessed for hypersensitivity, anemia, lupus erythematosus, methemoglobinemia, porphyria, rheumatoid arthritis, methemoglobin reductase deficiency, and glucose-6-phosphate dehydrogenase (G6PD) deficiency.
9. Mefloquine (Lariam) is indicated for the treatment of chloroquine-resistant malaria.
10. Each of these three patients has a protozoal infections. The patient with the intestinal disorder has giardiasis; the most likely drug treatment is metronidazole. The patient with AIDS has pneumocystosis; the most likely drugs for treatment include dapsone, atovaquone, primaquine, or clindamycin. The patient with the sexually transmitted infection has trichomoniasis; the most likely drug treatment is metronidazole.

Case Study

1. Intestinal roundworms are diagnosed based on symptoms and examination of stool specimens.
2. Contraindications to pyrantel (Combantin) include allergy to the medication and pregnancy. Even though Sandra is only 15 years of age, she should be assessed for possible pregnancy before this medication is given.
3. Based on Sandra's weight of 57 kg, the dose would be 627 mg (57 mg × 57 kg).

4. Pyrantel is generally well tolerated. The infrequent adverse effects are limited to vomiting and diarrhea. Headache, insomnia, irritability, drowsiness, dizziness, anorexia, abdominal cramps, nausea, and rash have also been reported.

CHAPTER 44
Antiseptic and Disinfectant Drugs

Critical Thinking Crossword

Across
1. Bactol
3. Nosocomial
4. aldehyde
6. betadine
7. iodine
9. Dakins

Down
2. Antiseptic
4. Acetic
5. Disinfectant
8. Lysol

Chapter Review

1. b, c, d
2. d
3. c
4. a
5. b
6. c

Case Study

1. The use of hydrogen peroxide as a solution to irrigate wounds is controversial. Its use may be detrimental to wounds because it can destroy newly forming cells as well as bacteria. In addition, tincture of iodine may stain the skin and cause irritation and pain at the site.
2. Dakin's solution is a sodium hypochlorite solution that may be used at 0.5% concentration for skin surfaces.
3. Sodium hypochlorite is also used in most household bleach solutions at 10.8% concentration or less and therefore has the characteristic bleach odour. The patient should be assured that Dakin's solution is a much weaker solution of sodium hypochlorite.
4. After the procedure, the nurse should wash her hands, dispose of contaminated dressings, record the nature of the procedure and findings, and maintain asepsis (surgical asepsis if the wound is open in any way or if the skin is not intact).

CHAPTER 45
Anti-Inflammatory, Antiarthritic, and Related Drugs

Chapter Review/Critical Thinking and Application

1. b
2. b
3. a, b, d
4. c
5. d
6. a
7. Symptoms of both salicylism (chronic salicylate intoxication) and acute salicylate overdose are similar, except that the effects are often more pronounced and they occur more quickly in the acute form. Acute salicylate overdose results from the ingestion of a single toxic dose. Chronic salicylate intoxication occurs as a result of either high doses or prolonged therapy with high doses.
8. Treatment of acute salicylate overdose consists of removing the salicylate from the gastrointestinal tract and preventing its absorption; correcting fluid, electrolyte, and acid–base disturbances; and implementing measures to enhance salicylate elimination.
9. Mr. Chesney has an acute overdose of a nonsteroidal anti-iflammatory drug (NSAID) that is not a salicylate. If the condition progresses, symptoms can include intense headache, dizziness, cerebral edema, cardiac arrest, and possibly death.
10. Treatment for Mr. Chesney will consist of removing the NSAID from the gastrointestinal tract followed by the administration of activated charcoal. Supportive and symptomatic treatment will be implemented. N-acetylcysteine is the antidote of choice for acetaminophen toxicity.
11. Mr. Henry needs to know that adherence to the entire medical regimen is important for the success of the treatment of gout. Allopurinol should be given with meals to help prevent the occurrence of gastrointestinal symptoms such as nausea, vomiting, and anorexia. Fluids should be increased to 3 L per day and hazardous activities should be avoided if dizziness or drowsiness occurs with the medication. Also, alcohol and caffeine should be avoided because these drugs will increase uric acid levels and decrease the levels of allopurinol.
12. Ketorolac (Toradol) is indicated for the short-term management (up to 5 days) of moderate to severe acute pain that requires analgesia at the opioid level. It is not indicated for minor or chronic pain.
13. The vinegary odour means that the Aspirin has experienced some chemical breakdown and she should not use it. She should discard it safely and purchase a new bottle.

Case Study

1. The specific COX-2 selectivity of these drugs allows them to control the inflammation and pain while not producing some of the toxicity associated with NSAID therapy.
2. The most common adverse effects include fatigue, dizziness, lower-extremity edema, hypertension, dyspepsia, nausea, heartburn, and epigastric discomfort. Report to the physician immediately any stomach pain, unusual bleeding, or blood in vomit or stool. Chest pain, palpitations, and any gastrointestinal problems should be reported as well.
3. Sadie should avoid alcohol and acetylsalicytic acid (Aspirin) while taking this medication and should check with her physician before taking any over-the-counter medications.

CHAPTER 46
Immunosuppressant Drugs

Chapter Review/Critical Thinking and Application

1. b
2. c
3. c
4. a
5. a, c, d
6. a
7. a. Daclizumab can help to prevent organ rejection. If Mrs. Flick's immune system cannot recognize the new heart as foreign, it will not mount an immune response against it.
   b. Laboratory studies should include hemoglobulin level, hematocrit, white blood cell count, and platelet count. These studies should be done before, during, and after therapy. If the leukocyte count drops below 3×10^9/L, the drug should be discontinued after the physician is notified.
   c. The antifungal drug is added several days before surgery as prophylaxis for *Candida albicans* infections.
8. Encourage the patient to take cyclosporine (Neoral) with meals or mixed with milk to prevent stomach upset.
9. Tess is experiencing symptoms consistent with adverse effects of muromonab-CD3.
10. Glatiramer acetate (Copaxone) is the only immunosuppressant drug that is currently indicated for the treatment of relapsing-remitting

multiple sclerosis. Glatiramer is used to reduce the frequency of relapses.

Case Study

1. Yes, immunosuppressant therapy will be lifelong.
2. White patches on the tongue, mucous membranes, and oral pharynx would be indicative of candidiasis.
3. Mr. Keller needs to be seen by a physician immediately. These symptoms could indicate that he has a severe infection.
4. If the leukocyte count drops below 3×10^9/L, then the drug should be discontinued because Mr. Keller is experiencing a severely immunosuppressed state.

CHAPTER 47
Immunizing Drugs and Pandemic Preparedness

Chapter Review/Critical Thinking and Application

1. a. Varicella vaccine
   b. Active
   c. Active
   d. *Haemophilus influenzae* type b prophylaxis
   e. Hepatitis B virus vaccine inactivated
   f. Rh_0 (D) immune globulin
   g. Passive
   h. Active
   i. Tuberculosis prophylaxis
   j. Active
   k. Diphtheria, tetanus, and pertussis prophylaxis, pediatric
   l. Passive
   m. Postexposure passive tetanus prophylaxis
   n. Active
   o. Diphtheria, tetanus, and acellular pertussis prophylaxis (adolescents)
2. b
3. d
4. a
5. a
6. c
7. Occasionally, after vaccination, the levels of antibodies against a particular pathogen decline over time and a second dose of the vaccine is given to restore the antibody titres to a level that can protect the person against the infection. This second dose is referred to as a *booster shot*.
8. Each year, a new influenza vaccine is developed that contains the three influenza virus strains that represent those strains that are likely to circulate in North America in the upcoming winter. The vaccination from the previous year

may not be effective for the influenza virus strains in the current year.
9. Jordan may experience localized swelling, redness, discomfort, and warmth at the injection site. Acetaminophen and rest are recommended for the relief of these adverse effects and the application of warm compresses to the injection site may also help to ease some of the discomfort.
10. Paul is experiencing more than the expected adverse effects of his vaccinations. He is probably experiencing "serum sickness," which may occur after repeated injections of equine-containing immunizing drugs. Because his symptoms may indicate respiratory impairment, he needs to be taken to the hospital for evaluation and monitoring. He may receive analgesics, antihistamines, epinephrine, or corticosteroids to treat this reaction.

Case Study

1. Rabies is a potent virus.
2. Those at high risk for rabies exposure, such as veterinarians, will receive the rabies virus vaccine (Imovox, Rabavert) as pre-exposure prophylaxis followed by booster shots based on blood titres. This is a type of active immunization.
3. As a volunteer, the nurse will receive drugs that give both active and passive immunization. Postexposure prophylaxis is given with injections of the rabies virus vaccine (see answer 2) and also with the rabies immune globulin (Imogam Rabies Pasteurized, Hyperrab). Because rabies can progress rapidly, the body has insufficient time to mount an adequate immune defense, and death occurs before it can do so. The passive immunization confers a temporary protection that is usually sufficient to keep the invading organism from causing death, even though it does not stimulate an antibody response. The active immunization will stimulate an antibody response.
4. The rabies virus vaccine will be given intramuscularly on the day of exposure (0) and on days 3, 7, 14, and 28, with one dose of rabies immune globulin within 7 days of the first vaccine dose. The rabies immune globulin is given as a single dose (20 units/kg); as much of the dose as possible is infiltrated into the bite wound area, and the remainder is given intramuscularly and not in the same injection site as the rabies vaccine.

CHAPTER 48
Antineoplastic Drugs Part 1: Cancer Overview and Cell Cycle–Specific Drugs

Critical Thinking Crossword

Across

1. Bifunctional
6. Emetic
9. Folic
11. Malignancy
12. Extravasation
13. Nadir

Down

2. Leucovorin
3. Benign
4. Leukemia
5. Spread
7. Alkylation
8. Mitosis
10. Limiting

Chapter Review

1. a, b, c, e, f
2. d
3. a
4. b
5. c

Case Study

1. Methotrexate is an antimetabolite, specifically, a folic acid antagonist. It inhibits the action of an enzyme that is responsible for converting folic acid to a substance used by the cell to synthesize DNA for cell reproduction. As a result, the cell dies.
2. Laboratory test results should be checked for white blood cell and red blood cell counts, hemoglobulin level and hematocrit, platelet counts, and renal and liver function studies.
3. The concurrent administration of nonsteroidal anti-inflammatory drugs (NSAIDs) and methotrexate may lead to severe bleeding tendencies. Allen should be instructed to avoid all NSAIDs, including acetylsalicylic acid (Aspirin), while taking methotrexate.
4. Antiemetic therapy and antacids are often needed to decrease nausea, vomiting, and gastrointestinal upset. Because methotrexate may cause hyperuricemia (increased uric acid levels) associated with tumour lysis syndrome, allopurinol (Alloprin, Zyloprim) may be given. Leucovorin may be used to protect the patient from potentially fatal bone marrow suppression, a toxic effect of methotrexate.

CHAPTER 49
Antineoplastic Drugs Part 2: Cell Cycle–Nonspecific and Miscellaneous Drugs

Chapter Review/Critical Thinking and Application

1. c
2. d
3. b
4. a, c, e, f
5. a
6. d
7. Cytoprotective drugs assist in reducing the toxicity of various antineoplastics. As a result, the adverse effects may be reduced or increased dosages of the antineoplastic medication may be tolerated, which allows greater cancer cell kill. For example, leucovorin and allopurinol can be used during therapy with methotrexate.
8. Mrs. Symthe should be assessed and monitored carefully for the development of pulmonary fibrosis and pneumonitis, which can occur during treatment with bleomycin (Blenoxane).
9. The nurse should not prepare the drug for infusion. In most facilities, institutional guidelines direct that the pharmacy department prepare these drugs. Special requirements must be met for the safety of those working with these drugs, including the use of a laminar airflow hood and appropriate personal protection equipment (e.g., gown, mask, and gloves). It would not be safe for the nurse or for those around the nurse to mix the chemotherapy drug on the nursing unit.
10. First, the nurse should stop the infusion immediately but not pull the catheter out. The physician should be notified immediately, and the nurse should expect to receive orders to treat the extravasation of mechlorethamine (Mustargen) by injecting a solution of 10% sodium thiosulfate and sterile water through the existing line into the extravasated site. The line can then be removed. Over the next few hours, Mr. Botolph will receive repeated subcutaneous injections into the area, and cold compresses should be applied to the site.

Case Study

1. Cisplatin is associated with nephrotoxicity, peripheral neuropathy, and ototoxicity.
2. Baseline renal studies should be performed, because the drug is highly nephrotoxic. If Dottie is receiving any other drugs that are potentially nephrotoxic, such as aminoglycoside therapy, dosage changes will need to be considered. If Dottie

has gout and is receiving treatment with probenecid (Benuryl) or sulfinpyrazone (Apo-Sulfinpyrazone), concurrent use of cisplatin may result in hyperuricemia or worsening of the gout. Baseline auditory studies should be performed, as well as baseline liver function studies and measurement of white blood cell count, hemoglobin level, hematocrit, and platelet level, because of the anticipated bone marrow suppression.

3. Because peripheral neuropathies may occur, numbness, tingling, or pain in the extremities should be reported to the physician immediately to prevent complications and enhance comfort.

4. This is a concern because dehydration while taking cisplatin may lead to kidney damage. Dottie should be reminded of the importance of hydration, and should be told to contact the physician if she experiences dry mucous membranes, dark amber urine or little or no urinary output, or vomiting of large amounts over a period of 8 hours or less. It may be a challenge, but Dottie needs to try to take in 3000 mL of fluid per day to prevent dehydration.

CHAPTER 50
Biological Response–Modifying Drugs

Chapter Review/Critical Thinking and Application

1. e
2. a
3. g
4. b
5. h
6. d
7. c
8. d
9. b
10. a, b, d, e
11. c
12. The major dose-limiting adverse effect of interferon is fatigue. Patients taking high dosages become so exhausted that they are often confined to bed. Sonja needs to know this before she starts the therapy.
13. Colony-stimulating factors (CSFs) such as filgrastim (Neupogen) and pegfilgrastim (Neulasta) can be given for chemotherapy-induced leukopenia. Thses drugs should be administered 24 hours after the chemotherapy drugs have been given because the myelosuppressive effects of the chemotherapy drugs tend to cancel out the therapeutic benefits of the CSFs.

14. Michiko will receive oprelvekin (Neumega), which is administered via subcutaneous injections daily for up to 21 days. Because Michiko has severe thrombocytopenia, however, the nurse must be careful to prevent excessive bleeding and bruising at the injection sites and to teach Michiko measures to reduce bleeding risks.

Case Study

1. Epoetin alfa (Epogen) is a synthetic derivative of the human hormone erythropoietin, which is produced primarily by the kidneys. It promotes the synthesis of erythrocytes (red blood cells) by stimulating the production of red blood cell precursors.
2. The hemoglobin level and hematocrit should be monitored carefully. If therapy is not halted when the target hemoglobulin of 120 g/L is reached or if the hemoglobin level and hematocrit rise too quickly, hypertension and seizures can result.
3. Epoetin is synthetically manufactured in mass quantities by means of recombinant DNA technology. This technology allows the drug to be essentially identical to its endogenously produced counterpart in the body.
4. Epoetin can be given either intravenously or subcutaneously. For administration at home, Connie will need to be taught subcutaneous administration.
5. Darbepoetin alfa (Aranesp) can be administered weekly, so the number of injections will obviously be less.

CHAPTER 51
Gene Therapy and Pharmacogenomics

Chapter Review/Critical Thinking and Application

1. g
2. f
3. b
4. c
5. d
6. DNA is deoxyribonucleic acid, located in the nucleus of all body cells as strands of chromosomes, collectively called *chromatin*. Protein synthesis is the primary function of DNA in the nuclei of human cells.
7. The goal of this scientific project was to map the entire DNA sequence (genome) of a human being.
8. The development of gene therapy and pharmacogenomics
9. Recombinant DNA is DNA that has been artificially synthesized or modified in a

laboratory setting. This technology is used to make recombinant forms of drugs such as hormones, vaccines, and antitoxins. The most common example of this technology is the use of the *Escherichia coli* genome so that these bacteria manufacture a recombinant form of human insulin.

10. The general goal of gene therapy is to transfer exogeneous genes to the patient, which will either provide a temporary substitute for or initiate permaneant changes in the patient's own genetic functioning to treat a given disease. Gene therapy techniques are being studied for the treatment of acquired diseases such as cancer, heart disease, and diabetes, but to date no gene therapy has received Health Canada approval for routine treatment of disease.

CHAPTER 52
Acid-Controlling Drugs

Chapter Review/Critical Thinking and Application

1. h
2. e
3. i
4. k
5. c
6. a, b
7. f
8. d
9. b
10. g
11. b
12. c
13. d
14. b, d, e
15. The nurses should inform Mr. Quang that long-term self-medication with antacids may mask symptoms of serious underlying diseases. He needs to be evaluated for possible bleeding ulcer or even a malignancy, but the nurse may not want to scare him with those possibilities. If his current self-treatment is no longer working, he needs a medical evaluation.
16. Omeprazole (Losec, Nexium) should be taken before meals and the entire capsule should be taken whole, not crushed, opened, or chewed. Omeprazole may also be given with antacids, if ordered. As with omeprazole, most of the proton pump inhibitors are given on a short-term basis, which should be emphasized to patients.
17. Patients with heart failure or hypertension should use antacids that are low in sodium. Mr. McKinney should also be told to take the antacid alone, not at the same time as other medications

(unless specifically instructed to do so), because the antacid will interfere with the absorption of the other medications. Antacids should be taken 1 hour before or 1 to 2 hours after other medications. If symptoms continue or worsen, he should consult his health care provider.

18. Antacids may promote premature dissolving of the enteric coating; if the coating is destroyed early in the stomach, gastrointestinal upset may occur. Mr. Wolowski should take the acetylsalicytic acid (Aspirin) tablets with food, not with antacids.

19. Frank will likely be placed on combination drug therapy referred to as *triple therapy*, which involves the use of a proton pump inhibitor such as lansoprazole (Apo-Lansoprazole) in addition to two different antibiotics, such as amoxicillin and clarithromycin, for 7 to 14 days. Often the recommended drug combinations are packaged together for convenience.

Case Study

1. Although histamine-2 (H$_2$) antagonists are available over the counter, the dose of the over-the-counter preparation is generally half the strength of the usual prescription dose.

2. The drug effects of H$_2$ blockers are limited to specific blocking actions on the parietal cells of the gastric glands in the stomach. As a result, hydrogen ion production is decreased, which leads to an increase in the pH of the stomach (i.e., decreased stomach acid).

3. The use of H$_2$ receptor antagonists is contraindicated in patients with known drug allergy or who have impaired kidney function or liver disease. Cautious use is recommended in patients who are confused or disoriented, or in older adults. Interactions may occur with drugs that have a narrow therapeutic range. Caution should be used if Eda is taking theophylline (Theolair) for her asthma. Patients requiring these medications should avoid acetylsalicylic acid (Aspirin) and other nonsteroidal anti-inflammatory drugs (NSAIDs), alcohol, and caffeine because of their ulcerogenic or gastrointestinal tract–irritating effects.

4. Smoking has been shown to decrease the effectiveness of H$_2$ blockers because the absorption of H$_2$ antagonists may be impaired in individuals who smoke. Hopefully, if Eda is not smoking, this will not be a problem for her, but spending several hours in a smoke-filled room may have an effect. Also, the beer and possibly spicy pizza may aggravate the underlying condition.

CHAPTER 53
Antidiarrheal Drugs and Laxatives

Critical Thinking Crossword

Across
1. Saline
4. Bulk-forming
7. Hyperosmotic

Down
2. Adsorbent
3. Anticholinergic
5. Emollient
6. Stimulant
8. Opiates

Chapter Review/Critical Thinking and Application

1. d
2. a
3. d
4. c
5. a, d
6. Darkening of the tongue or stool is a temporary and harmless adverse effect associated with bismuth subsalicylate (Pepto-Bismol).
7. The use of the belladonna alkaloid preparations, also known as anticholinergics, are contraindicated in patients with narrow-angle glaucoma. In Canada, belladonna is only available in combination with opium, so Mrs. Benedict's choices are limited even if she had no contraindications for this drug.
8. Several factors may be causing Hillary's constipation: lack of proper exercise, poor diet (which might involve inadequate roughage and an excess of dairy products), use of aluminum-containing antacids, and stress.
9. a. The bulk-forming laxatives tend to produce normal stools, have few systemic effects, and are among the safest available.
   b. Ira should mix the medication with at least 180 to 240 mL of fluid and drink it immediately. It should be taken alone (i.e., not with food) and is taken, as per the package insert instructions, usually in the morning and evening.
10. a. Because glycerin is mild, it is often used in children.
    b. Abdominal bloating and rectal irritation
11. a. It will probably be determined based on Kyle's weight.
    b. Kyle's mother should not give him any more medication, and she should contact the physician immediately.

Case Study

1. Antibiotic therapy destroys the balance of normal flora in the intestines and diarrhea-causing bacteria proliferate.
2. *Lactobacillus acidophilus* is indicated for diarrhea caused by antibiotic treatment that has destroyed the normal intestinal flora.
3. Exogenously supplying these bacteria helps restore the balance of normal flora and suppress the growth of diarrhea-causing bacteria.
4. It is considered a dietary supplement; it is often used for uncomplicated diarrhea, even though this is an off-label (non–Health Canada–approved) use.

CHAPTER 54
Antiemetic and Antinausea Drugs

Chapter Review/Critical Thinking and Application

1. a
2. c, e
3. d
4. c
5. b
6. Neuroleptic antiemetics. If Norman is taking levodopa for the Parkinson's disease, the beneficial effects of the levodopa could be reduced or cancelled because of a drug interaction with the neuroleptic drug.
7. a. Petra should take the metoclopramide 30 minutes before meals and at bedtime.
   b. Petra should be cautioned about taking the medication with alcohol because of the possible toxicity and central nervous system depression that can occur.
8. This drug is available in oral, intramuscular, intravenous, and rectal forms, but because Nellie is on "nothing-by-mouth" status and has no intravenous access, the intramuscular route was ordered. The nurses can call Nellie's physician for an alternate route, but the route cannot be changed without an order because the dosage may be different.
9. Dronabinol (Marinol) is a synthetic derivative of the major active substance in marijuana. You should explain to Chuck that dronabinol is used to stimulate appetite and weight gain in patients with AIDS.

Case Study

1. There are no significant drug interactions associated with the serotonin blockers such as ondansetron.

2. Antiemetics are often administered before a chemotherapy drug is given, frequently 30 minutes to 3 hours before treatment. Taking it only at the onset of nausea would have no useful effect.
3. Headache is caused by the ondansetron and can be relieved with acetaminophen.

CHAPTER 55
Pharmaconutrition

Critical Thinking Crossword

Across
1. erythromycin
4. Anabolism
5. Gastrostomy
8. Absorptive
10. Fatty acid
11. Essential
12. Nitrogen

Down
2. Catabolism
3. Enteral
6. Semiessential
7. Metabolism
8. Arginine
9. Phlebitis

Chapter Review/Critical Thinking and Application

1. a
2. c
3. a, c, d, e
4. c
5. a
6. d
7. a. Advantages of the newer tubes are that they are thinner and more pliable for better patient tolerance. However, they also make checking for gastric aspiration more difficult.
   b. If Ms. Schiller is lactose intolerant, she would experience cramping, diarrhea, abdominal bloating, and flatulence with the ingestion of lactose. In this case, lactose-free solutions should be used.
   c. The residual should not be more than 2 hours' worth of feeding, which in this case is no more than 100 mL. The nurse should return the aspirate, withhold the feeding, elevate the head of the bed, and notify the physician.
8. Mr. Robbins shows signs of fluid overload. The first thing the nurse should do is slow his infusion rate, then remain with him and contact the physician immediately. The nurse should continually assess his vital signs. Next time, the nurse can prevent this by maintaining intravenous rates, assessing the intravenous infusion every hour, and monitoring the patient's fluid status.

Case Study

1. If total parenteral nutrition is discontinued abruptly, rebound hypoglycemia may occur because the pancreas has not had time to adapt to the reduced blood glucose levels. Hypoglycemia is manifested by cold clammy skin, dizziness, tachycardia, and tingling of the extremities.
2. To prevent hypoglycemia, the nurse should hang a solution of 5% to 10% glucose to infuse until bag number 4 is ready. The nurse should also call to make sure the pharmacy is preparing the infusion bag.
3. During this infusion, Mrs. Thomas's blood glucose levels should be monitored on a regular basis. The nurse should assess for signs of hyperglycemia as well as hypoglycemia, signs of infection, and signs of fluid overload.

CHAPTER 56
Blood-Forming Drugs

Chapter Review/Critical Thinking and Application

1. d
2. b
3. c
4. a, b, c
5. b, c, d
6. d
7. Mr. Dlugy, who is about to receive his first dose of iron dextran, is at risk for fatal anaphylaxis. Because of this, a test dose of 25 mg of iron dextran should be administered by the chosen route and appropriate method of administration. An anaphylactic reaction should occur within a few moments, although waiting at least 1 hour before giving the rest of the initial dose is recommended. Intramuscular iron should be administered deep in large muscle mass using a Z-track method and a 23-gauge 4-cm needle.
8. Dietary sources of iron include meats and certain vegetables and grains. These forms of iron must be converted by gastric juices before thay can be absorbed. Other foods such as orange juice, veal, fish, and ascorbic acid may help with iron absorption. Conversely, eggs, corn, beans, and many cereal products containing chemicals known as *phytates* may impair iron absorption from other iron-containing foods or iron supplements. Both beans and eggs are common dietary sources of

iron. Antacids and milk products decrease the absorption of iron.

9. Treatment should include suction and maintenance of the airway, correction of acidosis, and control of shock and dehydration with intravenous fluids or blood, oxygen, and a vasopressor. Abdominal radiographs can allow visualization of the tablets. A serum concentration greater than 54 mmol/L will place David at serious risk for toxicity. Consultation with a Poison Control Centre is recommended. His stomach should be emptied immediately. Because many of the iron products are extended-release formulations that release their contents in the intestines rather than in the stomach, whole-gut irrigation using a polyethylene glycol solution is generally believed to be superior and more effective for decontaminating the bowel, followed by possible surgical removal of intake iron tablets.

10. A child with severe symptoms of iron intoxication will exhibit coma, shock, or seizures. Chelation therapy with deferoxamine should be initiated.

Case Study

1. Oral forms should also be given with juice (but not antacids or milk) between meals for maximal absorption. Should gastrointestinal distress occur, however, the iron can be taken with meals.

2. Maureen should be reminded that the use of any iron product will cause the stools to turn tarry and black.

3. Maureen should be told that one iron product cannot be substituted for another because each product contains different forms of the iron salt in different amounts.

4. Liquid oral forms of iron should be diluted per the manufacturer instructions and taken through a plastic straw to avoid discolouration of tooth enamel.

CHAPTER 57
Dermatological Drugs

Chapter Review/Critical Thinking and Application

1. a
2. b
3. a
4. b
5. a, b, d
6. d
7. The nurse would first ask Mr. Mugler about any allergies to other forms of drugs. If he has

an allergy to a particular antibacterial drug, that drug should not be used topically either. If culture and sensitivity testing is to be carried out, the specimen should be collected before the first application of the antibacterial drug. In this case, the nurse can apply a thin film of clindamycin (Clindasol Cream) and monitor for signs of allergy to clindamycin and other antibiotics.

8. Gloves are used not only to prevent contamination from secretions but also to prevent absorption of the medication through the skin of the person applying the medication.

9. Mr. Lacroix and his children are being treated for head lice. Tell him the following: "Leave the shampoo on for 4 minutes, then rinse and dry the hair. Then use a nit comb to remove nits (eggs) from the hair shafts." Other measures Mr. Lacroix should take include decontaminating the clothing and personal articles of the infested persons. All clothing, linens, stuffed toys, and other personal articles should be washed in hot soapy water or dry cleaned.

10. A patient taking any anti-acne drug should avoid ultraviolet light, weather extremes, sunlight, abrasive cleansers, and other keratolytic products. Sunscreen should be worn during therapy. Tretinoin (Retin-A) is available in many topical formulations, including creams, gels, and a liquid. Because of its potential to cause severe irritation and peeling, it may initially be applied once every 2 to 3 days, often starting with a lower-strength product. Benzoyl peroxide (Acetoxyl) generally produces signs of improvement in 4 to 6 weeks and adverse effects are infrequent and rarely a problem. Most adverse effects are confined to the skin and involve peeling of the skin, redness, or a sensation of warmth. Benzoyl peroxide is applied sparingly one to four times daily by lotion, gel, liquid, cleansing bar, moisturizer, or cream.

Case Study

1. Judy's allergies, especially any allergies to sulfonamide drugs, should be assessed. This cream should only be applied to areas that have been cleansed and debrided. The wound bed may need to be debrided before the cream can be applied.

2. The dressing helps keep the medication at the intended site and provides protection to the wound. In addition, it keeps the cream from soiling her clothing.

3. No. He should prevent contamination of the medication and avoid exposure to Judy's

wound secretions. He should apply the cream with a sterile, gloved hand.

4. The adverse effects of silver sulfadiazine are similar to those of other topical drugs and include pain, burning, and itching.

CHAPTER 58
Ophthalmic Drugs

Chapter Review/Critical Thinking and Application

1. c
2. h
3. j
4. k
5. a
6. d
7. b
8. f
9. g
10. e
11. c
12. b
13. b
14. d
15. b, c, d
16. c
17. The effect is less pronounced in individuals with dark eyes (brown or hazel) because pigment absorbs the drugs and dark eyes have more pigment than light eyes (blue).
18. a. Dipivefrin (Propine), a prodrug of epinephrine, has better lipophilicity than epinephrine and can penetrate into the anterior chamber of the eye. It is 4 to 11 times more potent than epinephrine in reducing intraocular pressure.
    b. Mrs. Ngo should report any stinging, burning, itching, lacrimation, or puffiness of the eye.
    c. No. Systemic effects are rare. They include cardiovascular effects and possibly headaches and faintness.
19. Ned may have had an allergic reaction to a preservative, such as benzalkonium chloride, in the first drug that was tried. Timolol is available in a preservative-free product.
20. a. Pilocarpine (Diocarpine) and carbachol (Miostat) can be used for Mrs. O'Rourke to reduce intraocular pressure associated with narrow-angle glaucoma. Pilocarpine and carbachol are cholinergic eye drops that cause miosis (constriction) of the pupil. This in effect pulls the peripheral iris away from the trabecular meshwork so that sometimes the aqueous humor can flow out of the eye through the meshwork and relieve the high intraocular pressure.

b. Headaches are an adverse effect of miotics.
21. The nonsteroidal anti-inflammatory drugs are considered less toxic, and they are preferred over the corticosteroids as initial topical therapy.
22. Stinging is normal after instillation of the drops; Ms. Luna should not wear her contact lenses while taking this medication.

Case Study

1. Ocular cytomegalovirus (CMV) infection is one of the many potential opportunistic infections associated with AIDS. Mr. Djukic did not contract the infection because he had poor hygiene; he was more susceptible to this infection because of his immunosuppressed condition.
2. Currently, the only treatment available in Canada is ganciclovir HCl (Valcyte), a tablet for oral treatment, and ganciclovir sodium (Cytovene) for intravenous infusion.
3. Ganciclovir sodium (Cytovene) is administered intravenously at 5 mg/kg every 12 hours, given as a constant intravenous infusion over 1 hour. Valcyte should be administered orally. The recommended dosage is 900 mg twice a day (with food).
4. Ganciclovir sodium (Cytovene) will be administered for 14 to 21 days. Valcyte is recommended to be taken for 21 days.

CHAPTER 59
Otic Drugs

Chapter Review/Critical Thinking and Application

1. a, b, d, e
2. d
3. b
4. a
5. c
6. The patient needs medical care immediately. His symptoms may be indicative of head trauma.
7. To take advantage of the steroidal anti-inflammatory, antipruritic, and antiallergic drug effects
8. a. Clean the ear, remove all cerumen by irrigation, and clean the dropper with alcohol. The drops also need to be at room temperature.
    b. André might become dizzy, so he should be supine when the drops are instilled.
9. a. The hydrocortisone will help to reduce the inflammation and itching associated with the infection.

b. A drug hypersensitivity or a perforated eardrum

10. Many ear disorders involve pain and inflammation. The anaesthetic effect of the local anaesthetic drugs makes them beneficial in treating these conditions.

11. a. The instructions are different for each boy. The pinna should be held up and back during instillation of ear drops in children older than 3 years of age, like Drew. For children 3 years of age and younger, like Ben, the pinna should be gently pulled down and back.
    b. Reduced pain, redness, and swelling are therapeutic effects of the medication.

12. a. Esther's husband should warm up the ear drops to body temperature by holding the bottle under warm running water, not soaking it in hot water, particularly because he should be careful to not let water get into the bottle or damage the label.
    b. Esther should not sit up right away. She should lie down on the side opposite the side of the affected ear for about 5 minutes after the drug is instilled. As an alternative, Esther can gently insert a small cotton ball into the ear canal to keep the drug in place, but the cotton ball should not be forced into the ear canal.

Case Study

1. Mark probably has an impaction of earwax in his ear canal. Such a buildup can cause pain and temporary deafness.

2. He should be taught that he should not insert anything in his ear canal. He will need to know how to clean his ears properly and how to use cerumen-removal drugs. The nurse may need to irrigate his ear canals before medication therapy is started.

3. This medication is given as otic (ear) drops. He will need to follow the manufacturer's recommendations for administration. He should lie on the side opposite the side of the affected ear for about 5 minutes after instillation of the drug. A small cotton ball may be inserted gently into the ear canal to keep the drug there, but it should not be forced into the ear or jammed down into the ear canal. When administering the drops, Mark should pull the pinna of his ear up and back.

4. Often, the simple application of olive or almond oil is sufficient to soften wax.

OVERVIEW OF DOSAGE CALCULATIONS

Introduction

Interpreting Medication Labels

1. Generic name: rifampin
   Trade name: Rifadin
   Unit dose: 300-mg capsule
   Total in container: 30 capsules
   Route: oral
2. Generic name: medroxyprogesterone acetate suspension
   Trade name: Depo-Provera
   Unit dose: 400 mg per mL
   Total in container: 2.5 mL
   Route: intramuscular use only

Section I

Basic Conversions Using Ratio and Proportion

1. 600,000 μg (mcg)
2. 1,500,000 μg (mcg)
3. 5 mg
4. 5000 mg
5. 2500 mg
6. 0.9 g (*Do not forget the leading zero.*)
7. 8000 g
8. 0.75 L (*Do not forget the leading zero.*)
9. 975,000 mL
10. 0.5 L (*Do not forget the leading zero.*)
11. 1.5 g
12. 20 mL
13. 12 tsp
14. 6 tbsp
15. 198 lb
16. 68.2 kg (*rounded to tenths*)
17. 24.2. lb

Section II

Calculating Oral Doses

1. 1 tablet
   0.5 g = 500 mg. Each tablet is 500 mg; therefore, 1 tablet is needed.
2. 2 tablets
   0.5 mg = 500 mcg
   250 mcg : 1 tablet :: 500 mcg : x tablet
   Proof: $250 \times 2 = 500$; $1 \times 500 = 500$
3. 0.5 tablet
   0.25 g = 250 mg
   500 mg : 1 tablet :: 250 mg : x tablet
   Proof: $500 \times 0.5 = 250$; $1 \times 250 = 250$
4. 20 mL
   12.5 mg : 5 mL :: 50 mg : x mL
   Proof: $12.5 \times 20 = 250$; $5 \times 50 = 250$

5. 4 mL
   0.1 g = 100 mg
   125 mg : 5 mL :: 100 mg : x mL
   Proof: 125 × 4 = 500; 5 × 100 = 500
6. 3 tablets
   0.3 g = 300 mg
   100 mg : 1 tablet :: 300 mg : x tablet
   Proof: 100 × 3 = 300; 1 × 300 = 300
7. 22.5 mL
   20 mEq : 15 mL :: 30 mEq : x mL
   Proof: 20 × 22.5 = 450; 15 × 30 = 450
8. 3 capsules
   0.15 g = 150 mg
   50 mg : 1 capsule :: 150 mg: x capsule
   Proof: 50 × 3 = 150; 1 × 150 = 150
9. 4 tablets
   2 g = 2000 mg
   500 mg : 1 tablet :: 2000 mg : x tablet
   Proof: 500 × 4 = 2000; 1 × 2000 = 2000

Section III

Reconstituting Medications

1. 2 mL
   100 mg : 1 mL :: 200 mg : x mL
   Proof: 100 × 2 = 200; 1 × 200 = 200
2. 1.5 mL
   40 mg : 1 mL :: 60 mg : x mL
   Proof: 40 × 1.5 = 60; 1 × 60 = 60
3. 0.8 mL
   10,000 units : 1 mL :: 8000 units : x mL
   Proof: 10,000 × 0.8 = 8000; 1 × 8000 = 8000
4. 1.5 mL
   500 mg : 1 mL :: 750 mg : x mL
   Proof: 500 × 1.5 = 750; 1 × 750 = 750
5. 20 mL
   125 mg : 5 mL :: 500 mg : x mL
   Proof: 125 × 20 = 2500; 5 × 500 = 2500
6. Choose the concentration using the 4.6-mL diluent. Using the 9.6-mL diluent would necessitate giving 3 mL intramuscularly versus the 1.5 mL using the 4.6-mL diluent.
   1.5 mL
   200,000 units : 1 mL :: 300,000 units : x mL
   Proof: 200,000 × 1.5 = 300,000; 1 × 300,000 = 300,000
7. 0.75 mL
   First: Convert mcg to mg : 750 mcg = 0.75 mg
   1:1000 indicates 1 g in 1000 mL, or 1000 mg in 1000 mL, or 1 mg/mL.
   1 mg : 1 mL :: 0.75 mg : x mL
   Proof: 1 × 0.75 = 0.75; 1 × 0.75 = 0.75
8. 1 mL
   NOTE: 1:5000 indicates 1 g in 5000 mL, or 1000 mg in 5000 mL, or 0.2 mg/mL.
   0.2 mg : 1 mL :: 0.2 mg : x mL

Proof: 0.2 × 1 = 0.2; 1 × 0.2 = 0.2
9. 9 mL
   NOTE: 10% indicates 10 g per 100 mL, or 0.1 g/mL.
   Need to ensure that units are alike: 900 mg = 0.9 g
   0.1 g : 1 mL :: 0.9 g : x mL
   Proof: 0.1 × 9 = 0.9; 1 × 0.9 = 0.9
10. 8 mL
    NOTE: 50% indicates 50 g per 100 mL, or 0.5 g/mL.
    0.5 g × 1 mL :: 4 g : x mL
    Proof: 0.5 × 8 = 4; 1 × 4 = 4

Section IV

Child Calculations

1. a. 0.46 to 47.3 mg/hr
      40 lb = 18.2 kg
      Low dose: 0.025 mg/kg/hr × 18.2 kg = 0.455, rounded to 0.46 mg/hr
      High dose: 2.6 mg/kg/hr × 18.2 kg = 47.32 rounded to 47.3 mg/hr
   b. Yes, the ordered dose of 1 mg/hr falls within the safe range for this child.
2. a. 75 to 150 mg/dose
      33 lb = 15 kg
      Low dose: 5 mg/kg/dose × 15 kg = 75 mg/dose
      High dose: 10 mg/kg/dose × 15 kg = 150 mg/dose
   b. 600 mg (40 mg × 15 kg = 600 mg/kg/24 hr)
   c. Yes, the ordered dose of 120 mg falls within the safe and therapeutic range for this child.
3. a. 3180 to 4770 mg/24 hr
      70 lb = 31.8 kg
      Low dose: 100 mg/kg/24 hr × 31.8 kg = 3180 mg/24 hr
      High dose: 150 mg/kg/24 hr × 31.8 kg = 4770 mg/24 hr
   b. 1060 to 1590 mg/dose
      Three doses in 24 hours; 3180 ÷ 3 = 1060 mg/dose; 4770 ÷ 3 = 1590 mg/dose
   c. No. 1.7 g = 1700 mg, which exceeds the safe dosage range for this drug for this child. (*Did you remember to convert grams to milligrams?*)
4. a. 0.14 to 0.36 mg/day
      15 lb = 6.8 kg
      Low dose: 0.02 mg/kg/day × 6.8 kg = 0.136, rounded to 0.14 mg/day
      High dose: 0.05 mg/kg/day × 6.8 kg = 0.34 mg/day
   b. 0.07 to 0.18 mg/dose
      "bid" doses are given twice in 24 hours.
      0.14 ÷ 2 = 0.07 mg/dose; 0.36 ÷ 2 = 0.18 mg/dose
   c. Yes, 150 mcg = 0.15 mg, which falls within the safe and therapeutic dose range for

this child. (*Did you remember to convert microgram (mcg) to milligrams (mg)?*)

5. a. 15.5 to 34.1 mg/kg/dose
   34 lb = 15.5 kg
   Low dose: 1 mg/kg/dose × 15.5 kg = 15.5 mg/dose
   High dose: 2.2 mg/kg/dose × 15.5 kg = 34.1 mg/dose
   b. Yes, the ordered dose of 30 mg is within the safe and therapeutic dose range for this child.

6. a. 60.8 to 76 mcg/kg/day
   50 lb = 22.7 kg
   Low dose: 4 mcg/kg/day × 15.2 kg = 60.8 mcg/day
   High dose: 5 mcg/kg/day × 15.2 kg = 76 mcg/day
   b. No. The ordered dose (0.2 mg = 200 mcg) exceeds the safe and therapeutic dose range for this child. (*Did you remember to convert micrograms to millilitres?*)

Section V

Basic Intravenous Calculations

1. Start at STEP 1. You need to calculate the hourly rate.
   a. 167 mL/hr
   1000 mL : 6 h :: x : 1 hr
   (1000 × 1) = (6 × x); 1000 = 6 x;
   x = 1000/6 = 166.66 (*Round to nearest whole number.*)
   Proof: 1000 × 1 = 1000; 6 × 167 = 1002
   (*slight difference due to previous rounding*)
   (Alternate method: 1000 mL ÷ 6 hr = 166.67 or 167 mL/hr)
   b. 42 gtt/min (*Round to nearest whole number.*)
   STEP 2:

   $\dfrac{\text{drop factor}}{\text{time (min)}} \times$ hourly rate = 15/60 × 167 = 1/4 × 200 = 41.75, rounded to nearest whole number

2. Start at STEP 1. You need to calculate the hourly rate.
   a. 200 mL/hr
   600 mL : 3 hr :: c : 1 hr
   (600 × 1) = (3 × x); 600 = 3 x;
   x = 600/3 = 200
   Proof: 600 × 1 = 600; 3 × 200 = 600
   (Alternate method: 600 mL ÷ 3 hr = 200 mL/hr)
   b. 33 gtt/min (*Round to nearest whole number.*)
   STEP 2:

   $\dfrac{\text{drop factor}}{\text{time (min)}} \times$ hourly rate = 10/60 × 200 = 1/6 × 200 = 33.33, rounded to nearest whole number

3. Start at STEP 1. You need to calculate the hourly rate.
   a. 83 mL/hr
   1000 mL : 12 hr :: x : 1 hr
   (1000 × 1) = (12 × x) ; 1000 = 12 x; x = 1000/12 = 83.33 (*Round to nearest whole number.*)
   Proof: 1000 × 1 = 1000; 12 × 83 = 996
   (*slight difference due to previous rounding*)
   (Alternate method: 1000 mL ÷ 12 hr = 83.33 or 83 mL/hr)
   b. 21 gtt/min (*Round to nearest whole number.*)
   STEP 2:

   $\dfrac{\text{drop factor}}{\text{time (min)}} \times$ hourly rate = 15/60 × 83 = 1/4 × 83 = 20.75, rounded to nearest whole number

4. Start at STEP 1. You need to calculate the hourly rate.
   a. 100 mL/hr
   200 mL : 2 hr :: x : 1 hr
   (200 × 1) = (2 × x); 200 = 2 x;
   x = 200/2 = 100
   Proof: 200 × 1 = 200; 2 × 100 = 200
   (Alternate method: 200 mL ÷ 2 hr = 100 mL/hr)
   b. 100 gtt/min
   STEP 2:

   $\dfrac{\text{drop factor}}{\text{time (min)}} \times$ hourly rate = 60/60 × 100 = 1 × 100 = 100

   c. The drop factor for microdrip tubing is 60 gtt/mL.

5. Start at STEP 2. The hourly rate has been provided (75 mL/hr).
   13 gtt/min (*Round to nearest whole number.*)
   STEP 2:

   $\dfrac{\text{drop factor}}{\text{time (min)}} \times$ hourly rate = 10/60 × 75 = 1/4 × 75 = 12.75, rounded to nearest whole number

6. Start at STEP 2. The hourly rate has been provided (75 mL/hr).
   19 gtt/min (*Round to nearest whole number.*)
   STEP 2:

   $\dfrac{\text{drop factor}}{\text{time (min)}} \times$ hourly rate = 15/60 × 75 = 1/4 × 75 = 18.75

7. Start at STEP 2. The hourly rate has been provided (75 mL/hr).
   19 gtt/min
   STEP 2:

   $\dfrac{\text{drop factor}}{\text{time (min)}} \times$ hourly rate = 20/60 × 75 = 1/3 × 75 = 25

8. As the drop factor increases, the drops per minute (gtt/min) also increase.

9. a. 100 mL/hr

b. and c. Since the infusion pump delivers in mL/hr, it is unnecessary to calculate drops per minute.

Start at STEP 1. You need to calculate the hourly rate. Remember, 30 min = 0.5 hr.

50 mL : 0.5 hr :: x mL : 1 hr

$(50 \times 1) = (0.5 \times x)$; $50 = 0.5\,x$;

$x = 50/0.5 = 100$

Proof: $50 \times 1 = 50$; $0.5 \times 100 = 50$

(Alternate method: 50 mL ÷ 0.5 hr = 100 mL/hr)

10. Start at STEP 1. You need to calculate the hourly rate.
   a. 125 mL/hr

   500 mL : 4 hr :: x : 1 hr

   $(500 \times 1) = (4 \times x)$; $500 = 4\,x$;

   $x = 500/4 = 125$

   Proof: $500 \times 1 = 500$; $4 \times 125 = 500$

   (Alternate method: 500 mL ÷ 4 hr = 125 mL/hr)

   b. 125 gtt/min

STEP 2:

$$\frac{\text{drop factor}}{\text{time (min)}} \times \text{hourly rate} = 60/60 \times 125 = 1 \times 125 = 125$$

Practice Quiz

1. 0.75 mg

   1000 mcg : 1 mg :: 750 mcg : x mg

   Proof: $1000 \times 0.75 = 750$; $1 \times 750 = 750$

2. 8000 mg

   1 g : 1000 mg :: 8 g : x mg

   Proof: $1 \times 8000 = 8000$; $1000 \times 8 = 8000$

3. 113.6 kg

   1 kg : 2.2 lb :: x kg : 250 lb

   Proof: $1 \times 250 = 250$; $2.2 \times 113.6 = 249.92$

   (rounds to 250)

4. 165 lb

   1 kg : 2.2 lb :: 75 kg : x lb

   Proof: $1 \times 165 = 165$; $2.2 \times 75 = 165$

5. 15 mL

   1 tsp : 5 mL :: 3 tsp : x mL

   Proof: $1 \times 15 = 15$; $5 \times 3 = 15$

6. 10 mL

   25 mg : 5 mL :: 50 mg : x mL

   Proof: $25 \times 10 = 250$; $5 \times 50 = 250$

7. 1 tablet

   STEP 1: Convert grams to milligrams:

   0.5 g = 500 mg

   500 mg : 1 tablet :: 500 mg : x tablet

   Proof: $500 \times 1 = 500$; $1 \times 500 = 500$

8. 2 mL

   50 mg : 1 mL :: 100 mg : x mL

   Proof: $50 \times 2 = 100$; $1 \times 100 = 100$

9. 5 mL

   1% indicates 1 g in 100 mL, which equals 1000 mg/100 mL, or 10 mg/1 mL.

   10 mg : 1 mL :: 50 mg : x mL

   Proof: $10 \times 5 = 50$; $1 \times 50 = 50$

10. 0.25 mL

    1:1000 indicates 1 g in 1000 mL, which equals 1000 mg/1000 mL, or 1 mg/mL.

    1 mg : 1 mL :: 0.25 mg : x mL

    Proof: $1 \times 0.25 = 0.25$; $1 \times 0.25 = 0.25$

11. 1.5 mL

    10,000 units : 1 mL :: 15,000 units : x mL

    Proof: $10,000 \times 1.5 = 15,000$; $1 \times 15,000 = 15,000$

12. a. 0.2 mg/dose
    b. Yes, the dose of 1 mg does not exceed the safe and therapeutic dosage range for this child.

    22 lb = 10 kg

    Acceptable range: 0.2 mg/kg/dose × 10 kg = 2 mg/dose

13. a. 63 mL/hr

    500 mL ÷ 8 hr = 62.5, rounded to 63 mL/hr

    b. 16 gtt/min

    $$\frac{\text{drop factor}}{\text{time (min)}} \times \text{hourly rate} = 15/60 \times 63 = 1/4 \times 63 = 15.75, \text{rounded to nearest whole number}$$

14. a. Infusion pumps deliver mL/hr.
    b. 50 mL/hr (as stated in the question)

15. a. 42 mL/hr

    1000 mL ÷ 24 hr = 41.67, rounded to 42 mL/hr

    b. 42 gtt/min (*Remember, if the drop factor is 60, the rate is the same as the drops per minute (gtt/min).*)

    $$\frac{\text{drop factor}}{\text{time (min)}} \times \text{hourly rate} = 60/60 \times 42 = 1 \times 42 \text{ gtt/min}$$

16. a. 750 mg
    b. 5.6 mL

    90 mg : 1 mL :: 750 mg : x mL

    Proof: $90 \times 5.6 = 500$; $1 \times 500 = 500$

17. a. 200,000 units/mL
    b. 23 mL
    c. 1 mL (concentration is 200,000 units per 1 mL)
    d. Label the multidose vial with the date, time, amount of diluent used, and user's initials.

18. a. 6 mL

    100 mg : 1 mL :: 600 mg : x mL

    Proof: $100 \times 6 = 600$; $1 \times 600 = 600$

    b. Up to 1410 mg/24 hr

    31 lb = 14.1 kg; 14.1 kg × 100 mg/kg/day = 1410 mg/24 hr (safe dose)

    c. 705 mg/dose

    There are two doses per day; 1410 mg ÷ 2 = 705 mg/dose

    d. Yes

    The ordered dose of 600 mg does not exceed the 705 maximum dose.

19. 2.5 mL

    125 mcg = 0.125 mg

    0.05 mg : 1 mL :: 0.125 mg : x mL

    Proof: $0.05 \times 2.5 = 0.12502$ $1 \times 0.125 = 0.125$

Notes